# CHRIS MARCO FLORES

# THE WEIGHT IS OVER

## How to escape the body that you feel trapped in

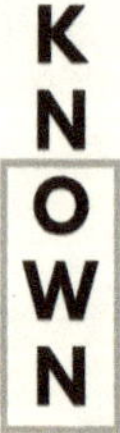

www.get-known.co.uk

# CONTENTS

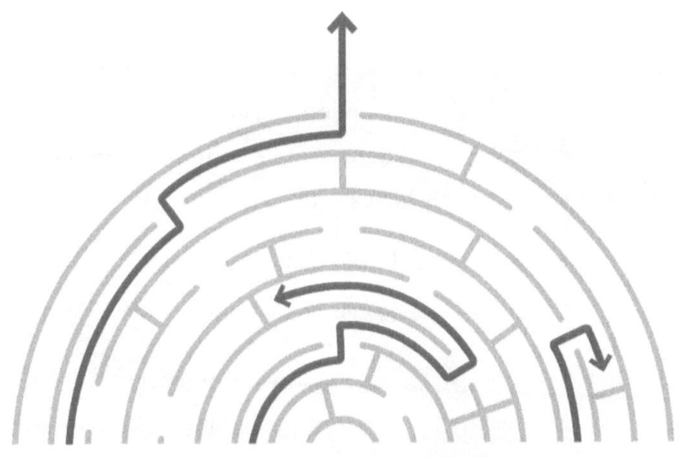

# INTRODUCTION

## WEALTH + HEALTH = HAPPINESS

Imagine there are two sides to life. The left side is the sad side of life, and the right side is the happy side of life. The further to the left side of life you are, the harder it feels to get back over to the right and the more trapped and sadder you become. This triggers depression, anxiety, stress and even suicidal thoughts. The further to the right side, the freer you feel and the happier you become. This triggers joy, contentment, pleasure, freedom, well-being, satisfaction and contentment with life.

There are two aspects that you will 100% need to keep you on the right side of life and ensure you have the freedom you need to stay away from the caged life (left side).

A level of wealth because everyone needs a certain amount to be able to live the life they desire. This will mean different things to different people. Some people want to be millionaires and others are perfectly happy with far less.

A level of health because health is the real wealth and without health, it's very hard to enjoy anything in life.

If you are rich but suffering from health problems, or if you are perfectly healthy but impoverished you will find yourself trapped on the sad side of life. If you are poor and have health problems then you will find life a struggle. In any of these scenarios, the longer you stay in that position, the worse it will get and the more you start to believe that your life will never get any better. It's a slippery slope, trust me!

However, this doesn't have to be the case. I have worked with many people who have completely turned their health and lives around. In this book, I want to empower you to do the same, no matter what your starting point is or what change you want to make. This book will give you the foundation that you need to help you escape an unhealthy, overweight body. It will give

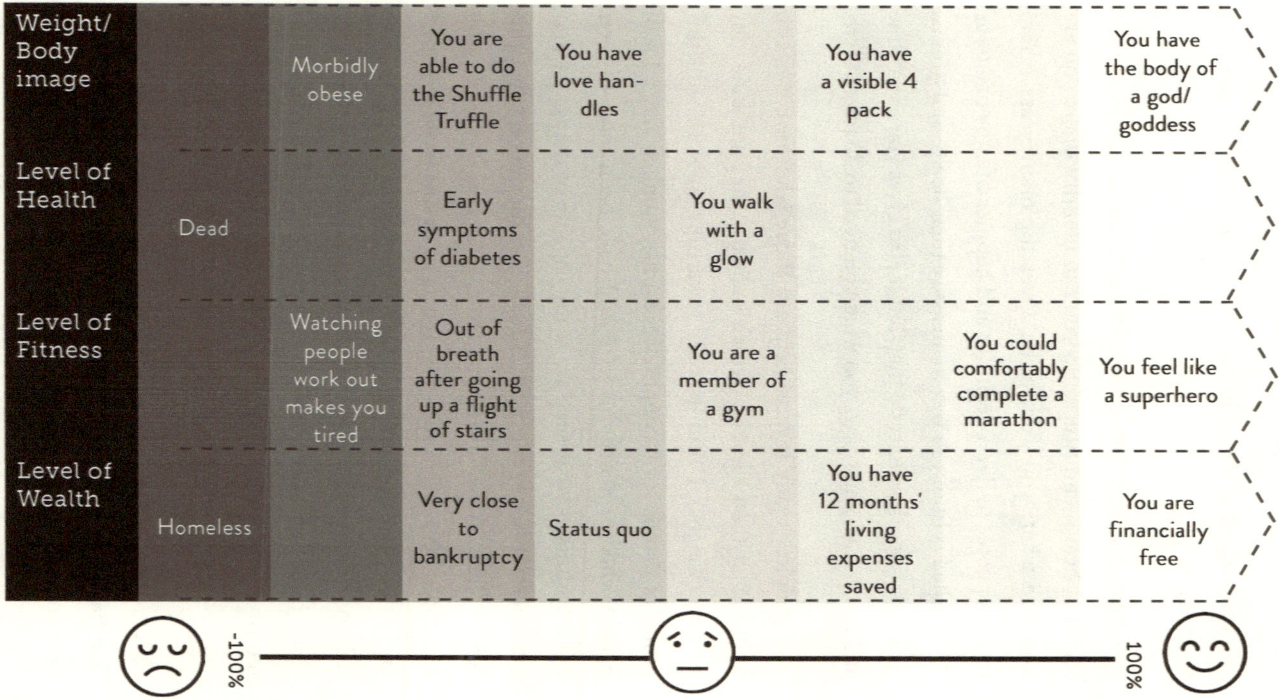

| | | | | | | | |
|---|---|---|---|---|---|---|---|
| **Weight/ Body image** | Morbidly obese | You are able to do the Shuffle Truffle | You have love han-dles | | You have a visible 4 pack | | You have the body of a god/ goddess |
| **Level of Health** | Dead | Early symptoms of diabetes | | You walk with a glow | | | |
| **Level of Fitness** | Watching people work out makes you tired | Out of breath after going up a flight of stairs | | You are a member of a gym | | You could comfortably complete a marathon | You feel like a superhero |
| **Level of Wealth** | Homeless | Very close to bankruptcy | Status quo | | You have 12 months' living expenses saved | | You are financially free |

-100%      100%

you motivation, hope, guidance and actions that you can start taking today.

I've created a chart (below) to show you the various levels and scales of health and fitness, so you can identify where you are now and where you want to be. Over the many years I have trained people to live a healthier and happier life, the one issue they've had is finding a way to measure their health and fitness. Not only does this chart do that, but it also gives you a start line and finish line, and shows you what you need to do to get there.

The people I really love to help are those who have a health level higher than a level 5 (which indicates they are unhealthy and overweight). I find it really rewarding to work with this group of people for a couple of reasons. Number one, a lot of people who are above a level 5 and have been most of their life are blind to what they are really capable of doing. As they have been this way for most of their life, they accept that this is how their life will always be. However, when I speak to a lot of people who are in this position they desire to be healthier and fitter than they are and there is no better feeling than to help people to pull the curtain back and push them to achieve something they never thought was possible, which is a health-ier, fitter and happier life. This leads me on to reason number two: I believe these people need the help the most.

Often, they spend most of their lives achieving great things, like having a successful career and bringing up their family, and end up looking after everything else in their lives apart

# FITNESS & HEALTH

## Level Scale

## LEVEL OF HEALTH

Out of the 7 Levels of HEALTH, tick one that best applies to you

| MEN | WOMEN | LEVEL OF HEALTH | ☑ |
|---|---|---|---|
| 30+% | 40+% | Level 7: Super Overweight | |
| 27-30% | 30-40% | Level 6: Overweight | |
| 23-26% | 27-29% | Level 5: Fat | |
| 18-22% | 23-26% | Level 4: Chubby - healthy | |
| 14-17% | 19-22% | Level 3: Healthiest | |
| 6-13% | 16-18% | Level 2: Healthy - Toned body | |
| 2-5% | 12-15% | Level 1: Dangerously low body fat | |
| <2% | <12% | Level 0: Extremely dangerous | |

## LEVEL OF FITNESS

Out of the 7 Levels of FITNESS, tick one that best applies to you

| FITNESS TESTS | S&C TEST | ENDURANCE 10K TEST | ACTIVITY | ☑ |
|---|---|---|---|---|
| Athlete fit | 300+ | 40 mins or less | Flyer | |
| Super fit | 300 | 40- 45 mins | Sprinter | |
| Healthy fit | 270 | 45 - 50 mins | Runner/Jumper | |
| Fit | 250 | 60-90 mins | Runner | |
| Unfit | 200 | 120 mins | Jogger | |
| Very unfit | 180 | 120 + mins | Walker | |
| Extreme unfit | 140 | Didn't Complete | Crawler | |

MY FITNESS LEVEL ▶ [　]   MY HEALTH LEVEL ▶ [　]

from their health. Their health had become the last thing on their list of priorities, and before they know it, they are either a size 22 (if they are a woman) or a trouser size 40 (if a man).

No matter where you find yourself on this chart, by using my system you will get to a healthy weight.

As we go through this book, I will be motivating and encouraging you to improve your health and fitness. If you have never done any fitness work in your life and/or you have any concerns about it, please check with your GP to make sure it is okay for you to start undertaking physical activity. As you read on, you will find that my process is a gradual one, so you won't be thrown in at the deep end. Nevertheless, if there is anything you are unsure about, please check it with your GP.

The higher you go up the health table the more you are putting your health at risk. As soon as you hit level 5 you want to make it your number 1 priority to get back into the healthier levels. Once you are at a level 7 (dangerously overweight) you are at risk of having irreversible health conditions. Always remember this saying, "Prevention is better than cure."

If you want to change, it is up to you. It takes bravery and courage to admit you have a problem, but no matter where you are on the scale, it's time to make your health your number 1 priority. You owe that to yourself and your family.

Let me tell you first-hand, your health is the most important aspect of your life. Even Steve Jobs said on his death bed, "I have more money than most people can imagine, but right now, all I want is my health and my family."

Every single one of us is built to move, walk, run, jump, climb and if you are physically capable of being able to move, then you should take as much advantage of this opportunity as you can, because you never know when you will have it taken away from you. Yes, some people can do it better than others, but you wouldn't ask a fish to climb a tree, because it would be physically impossible, that's not what a fish is designed for. A human is not designed to sit down all day every day, even though it is possible for a human to do so. However, that is what a lot of people do and thereby fail to use their bodies to their full potential.

People can give you money, cars, and even houses if you are lucky enough, but no one can give you your health. Your health is something you need to create for yourself and to do so, you have to change not just your diet but your lifestyle, and that could even mean changing the people you hang around with.

I'm going to help you adopt a healthier attitude. Instead of spending money on a night out, you will be spending money on a gym membership and fitness clothes. Instead of booking a holiday, you will spend the money on a weight-loss programme. Instead of spending the evening drinking a couple of cocktails or beers with your friends, you will use that time to prepare your food for the next day or week ahead, or if you have already

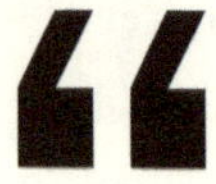

THIS JOURNEY CAN BE VERY ENJOYABLE, BUT YOU NEED TO UNDERSTAND THAT YOUR PRIORITIES MUST CHANGE FOR YOU TO CHANGE.

done this, use the time to go for a walk, cycle or swim, or take part in another fitness session to help you burn off some extra calories. You will do this until you have got yourself into the position that you want to be in.

You might think that doesn't sound like fun and won't allow you to enjoy your life, but remember that health is an important part of the happiness equation. So what would you rather do, spend 12 months being disciplined, making your health a priority and doing all the things I have just mentioned, so that you can live in a healthy body that makes you feel amazing and gives you the confidence to do whatever you want for the rest of your life, or spend the rest of your life in a body that makes you miserable, on yoyo diets that can't give you the long-lasting results you desire and need? This journey can be very enjoyable, but you need to understand that your priorities must change for you to change.

## ARE YOU READY FOR THE WEIGHT IS OVER?

If you are sitting there reading this and thinking that you can't get the results because you are too overweight and think fitness is not for you, or you feel forever caged in a body you do not know how to escape from, let me tell you that things can change. I have created a proven route that will help you to improve both your level of health and physical fitness, regardless of your situation. It will set you free and make you feel fearless towards life. It's called The Weight is Over, Making the Impossible; Possible. This is a 12-month programme that takes you through a series of exercise and nutrition methods that will not only change your life forever, but also help you identify which nutrition and exercise methods will work best for you and your lifestyle.

In this book, I am going to teach you the The Weight is Over methods that I used to help over 40 people lose 100+ stone (1,400lbs) within the 6 months that it took me to write this book.

Is it easy? Absolutely not. Is it simple? Yes! If you persist and do not chuck the towel in, it will change your life forever. Just like it did mine and the many others I have helped. Just remember that anything great in life is not easy.

With my The Weight is Over method, not only will you break free from a body you feel trapped in but also become fearless towards life. You will become fearless about tackling any physical challenge put your way and, most importantly, your mind will be fearless when facing any life challenge, whether it is happily standing in front of a camera and having your photo taken or getting dressed up to go out on a night out. You will be filled with confidence. You will be able to look back and know that you have done it with pride!

How do you break free? Everyone works in different ways. I'm going to show you the method I have created, which has worked over and over again for my clients. If you follow this method you will gain nothing but success.

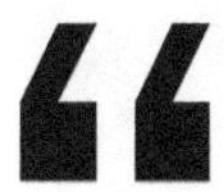

ONE OF THE BIGGEST REASONS

WHY PEOPLE FAIL TO ACHIEVE

A HEALTH AND FITNESS GOAL

IS THEY DO NOT DO THEIR

HOMEWORK AND JUMP TOO FAR

IN AT THE DEEP END. YOU MUST

LAY THE FOUNDATIONS FIRST.

# THE THE WEIGHT IS OVER WAY

The Weight is Over has 8 missions: If you would like to know more about the purpose of these missions you can go to my website www.chrismarcoflores.com

1.  Unlock

2.  Believe

3.  Achieve

4.  Escaping Shallow Hal

5.  Fight the fear

6.  Turn the Impossible to Possible

7.  Remember and realise

8.  Freedom, Fearless & Pride

Each mission has a purpose and an aim so that you can understand why you need to do what you need to do. For you to understand each mission in-depth, it would require me to write another book on its own (which is what I will be doing after I have finished writing this one). I have given a short explanation of the first mission later on in this book, so you can get an idea of how important it is, as well as the purpose, which is to help you escape the unhealthy, overweight body that you feel trapped in.

# THE 5 VITAL ACTIVITIES

Each mission takes 6 weeks to complete and is broken down into 5 Vital Activities. These Vital Activities form a stepping stone to getting the mission completed. Each one is very important and needs to be given careful attention and the time that is necessary to implement it before moving on to the next. It's a process that can be applied to any physical challenge in life. This 5-step strategy (5 Vital Activities) will help you with any challenge or mission that you experience with your health and fitness. I take myself through this process before I take on any physical challenge. Whenever I take on a new client, this process is the first thing I will take them through, regardless of their goal. Below is a list of the 5 Vital Activities that I will explain in detail in this book:

1. Mindset

2. Challenge

3. Exercise

4. Nutrition

5. Plan & Prepare

In this book, I will cover each of the 5 Vital Activities and explain how you can use them to start your journey to becoming healthier, fitter and happier. Even if you don't think it is possible, I will show you how. I will also share my story with you about how I achieved things I didn't even know were possible,

> YOU HAVE TO LEARN WHAT MAKES YOU KEEP PUTTING THE WEIGHT ON AND WHICH METHOD WORKS BEST FOR YOU AND YOUR BODY.

which gave me the motivation to do what I am doing now. I am also going to share with you some of my clients' stories and explain what we have done to help change their lives. This will help you if you are in the same position as they once were.

One of the biggest reasons why people fail to achieve a health and fitness goal is they do not do their homework and jump too far in at the deep end. You must lay the foundations first.

For example, let's say Jill Bloggs is a size 22 and wants to lose weight and eat healthily. She decides to start doing some sort of exercise, starting the following Monday. What tends to happen with people like Jill, who have no plan, aim, purpose, timescale, direction or defined goal, is they fall at the first hurdle.

Structure is the most important part of the whole process. Achieving your health and fitness goal is like building a pyramid. The 5 Vital Activities are the 5 solid foundation stones. If you do not have one of the Vital Activities properly in place, then it's impossible to lay the next level. That's how serious you need to be to take these next steps if you truly want to successfully achieve your desired goal. In the latter part of this book, there is a chapter on each of these 5 Vital Activities, clearly explaining what they are, why they are important and how you can start utilising them. There will be activities for you to do as well as plenty of things for you to think about.

# WHY THIS TIME WILL BE DIFFERENT

Using the 5 Vital Activities, I helped a client of mine called Andrew, who had been stuck at a weight he could not escape, lose a total of 9 stone, a result he didn't think was possible.

If you do not break the back of the task, you will always be trapped in an unhealthy, overweight body.

To achieve this you must not stop until you have hit the point of no return. For example, it's great to lose 3 stone, but if you need to lose 5, you haven't finished your journey. First, you have to break the habits that you may have created over the years.

A lot of people create a long-lasting pattern which is also a very bad habit. They will start a diet, do it for a couple of weeks or a few months, lose a little or a lot of weight and feel great. Their confidence grows and then they stop the diet and go back to their original lifestyle. Then, over time, they put it all back on. So, they start another diet or programme, lose some more weight and then once again, put it back on and this will happen throughout their life. It's an exhausting cycle I want you to get out of.

You have to learn what makes you keep putting the weight on and which method works best for you and your body.

Knowing this will help you to shed that fat and keep it off. This is not about what works best for Karen down the road. What might work for Karen might not work for you.

If you feel like you are on the left side of the scale then start taking action (taking action is going to be your new best friend).

Your first challenge is to start reading this now. Not tomorrow or next Monday. Start changing your life right now, this very second.

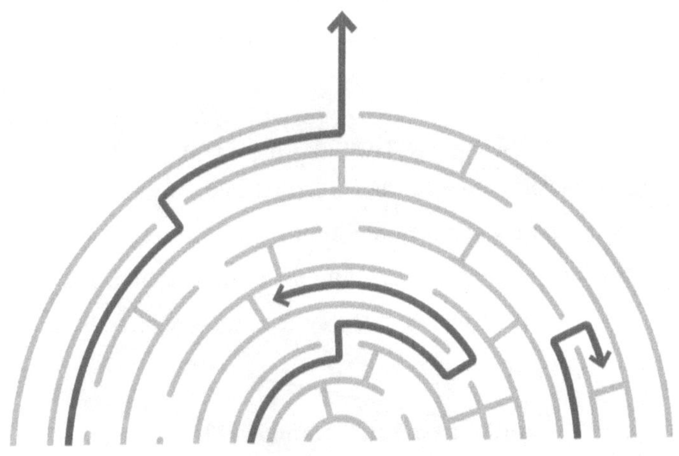

# MY STORY

My name is Chris Marco Flores and I was once caged in an unhappy body. I did not enjoy looking at myself, my health was non-existent and fitness was not my friend. I have always been an outwardly happy person, but behind the smiles and joy, I felt worthless. I grew up just thinking and accepting that was how my life would always be.

# 3 MAJOR THINGS THROUGHOUT MY LIFE JOURNEY CHANGED ME:

1. **Joining the British Army** – The British Army (Coldstream Guards) was my first major life event. Within just 6 months, I became barbarically fit, but it came with a price because I thought I knew everything.

2. **Joining the American Army** – I continued my development in the US Army, where I was an infantry airborne soldier (yes, I have served in two armies). This opened up my mind and helped me to think outside of the systematic way I had been programmed.

3. **Becoming a personal trainer** – This enabled me to put everything I had learned to use and help other people, which is immensely rewarding. As well as developing my understanding of the science behind fitness, I learned how important it is to work smarter instead of harder. It also taught me that you are forever learning in life and should never stop trying to learn!

These three major events have helped me to understand how health and fitness saved my life. I will share more details about these events throughout the book. Thankfully, these tough events I put myself through have changed my life, like I could never have imagined. From being incredibly unfit and feeling unworthy, I managed to reach a point where I am so physically and mentally fit that I fear no challenge. Now I know how to get my mind and health to a position where I feel on top of the world.

When I see people who are suffering due to their health, I know I can help them escape and turn the impossible to the possible. And if I had all the money in the world, that is what I would spend my time doing – changing people's lives.

## THE UNHEALTHIEST KID IN SCHOOL

Before I joined the British Army at a very young age, I was extremely unfit. I could never finish a school rugby match and would always pretend to hobble off the pitch injured before half-time because my fitness was so poor.

A lot of my friends went to the local boxing club and I didn't want to be left out so I joined them. Before we would start a boxing session, they made us warm-up with a long run (1-5 miles) and most times I would just run (hobble) home. Again, because of my lack of fitness, the embarrassment was unbearable.

Our school cross-country course used to be one big loop, and the first time I ran it, I got back so late that most of the other students were showered and dressed. After that, every time I did cross-country, I ran until we were out of sight and then jumped into a bush to hide. I would then wait for them to come back, before jumping out and joining the group again.

I could have easily won an award for the most unfit kid in the school and to make it worse I had no interest in fitness.

I wasn't obese, I was the opposite. I was very underweight and found it impossible to put weight on to the point that I remember when I was 14 years old my cousin told me to put a shirt on because my bony body was putting her off her food.

If being the unhealthiest kid in school wasn't bad enough, I also used to suffer from acne. It was so bad that I would wake up and the sheets of my bed would be covered in blood because the spots would pop by themselves. I was completely covered in pimples, which was a source of misery throughout my teenage years and really affected my confidence. This unhappiness and feeling of being worthless lasted throughout my school years, and I even found it very hard to speak to girls because I didn't feel like I was worthy enough.

On top of that, there was always someone who wanted to pick on me or beat me up for some reason. I can't put my finger on why, but I imagine it was due to the colour of my skin. I am a quarter Mexican and a quarter Indian and the rest of me is British. There weren't many people in my town with dark skin like mine. For whatever reason, I was targeted and beaten up a lot until I started fighting back.

School was a hard 5 years for me.

## 1. BRITISH ARMY TRAINING – getting seriously fit for the first time

Once I finished school, I didn't really have any sense of direction. I was a bit of a sheep (which, in this instance, was an advantage) and all my friends wanted to join the Army. Initially, the thought of joining the Army was just a big fat NO in my mind. I thought my friends were all crazy. However, they all started going through the procedure of entering the Army recruitment office and, of course, I came along with them.

When I was in the Army office, the Army Recruiting Sergeant who was from the Coldstream Guards started to talk to me. He asked about my life and if I had ever thought about joining and what it could do for me.

I remember sitting there, wondering why the recruiting sergeant was talking to me and even considering me – a skinny, spotty 15-year-old boy – as being worthy of joining his Army. I felt privileged that this guy, who I had massive respect for in an army uniform, would even talk to me, let alone entertain the thought that I could join the Army.

As he spoke, he made me feel, for the first time in my life, that this could be something that I felt proud to be a part of. It was the first opportunity I'd had to prove to myself that I was worthy of something in life.

I went through the recruitment process, and ironically, I was the only one out of all my friends who completely signed up.

It took me about a year to join. It gave me a sense of purpose, a focus and a big enough reason to start thinking about increasing my fitness and health level.

Before I knew it, I was officially in the British Army and joining a regiment called the Coldstream Guards. Before we could join the regiment, we had to undergo 6 months of basic training. It is basically a 6-month interview because if you are not good enough by the end of this period, you cannot join the regiment. In my eyes, it is by far the toughest job interview on the planet.

This was the toughest 6 months of my life, but it was also the most rewarding. A total of 55 people signed up but only 17 managed to complete the training because it was that hard. (Ironically, my platoon was called 17 Platoon, which is another book on its own.)

Throughout these 6 months, they broke me down. I tried to quit 3 times and I packed my bags twice to run away because it was so mentally and physically demanding I wanted to quit. Thankfully, I got through it, and doing so helped to shape me into the man I am today by laying the foundations.

I became mentally and physically fit. It was my first taste of how great true health felt. My mind was unlocked and I felt like I could take on the world.

After 6 months, I went home fitter than anyone I knew. I went back to the boxing club and I was the first person back from the warm-up run. I went down to the local rugby club and was running rings around all players due to my fitness. I was a new man, full of confidence. I looked good and I felt on top of the world!

It did come with a drawback, however, because I became so fit I thought I knew everything. I no longer wanted to listen to anyone else, no matter how knowledgeable they were, when it came to health and fitness. If I wanted a six-pack, I would do 300 sit-ups every day until I got one. This is the barbaric method. But that 6 months had installed a drive and desire inside me to better my life in every single way.

## 2. US ARMY TRAINING – discovering a passion for fitness and testing myself in new ways

When I left the British Army in 2008, I felt lost. I didn't know what to do with my life. I'd always had the ambition to join the American army as an infantryman and my dream was to join the Special Forces. It took me 2 years to build up the courage to move over to America and try to join.

At the age of 20, I moved to Washington State to try and enlist in the US Army, and I came up against a lot of hurdles (to put it lightly). It took me until the age of 21 to be an infantryman, and I could write a book about my journey through the two armies and the hurdles that I had to overcome to join them, which I will one day.

THERE ARE 24 HOURS IN
THE DAY AND I THANK THE US
ARMY FOR TEACHING
ME HOW TO UTILISE THEM.

But what I want to talk about in this book is how, during the 5 years prior to joining the American army, I dedicated a lot of time to improving my fitness. I became incredibly fit. To give you a little idea of how fit I was, I trained four hours a day, six days a week.

They have a fitness test throughout your Army career with a measurable score, with 300 being the maximum score you can get. I scored a 300 before the US Army training began, you couldn't get any higher. I also had years of British army training and experience. I was in excellent shape and ready for the challenge.

I was finally accepted into the US Infantry and I remember the first day I was dropped off at the recruitment centre by my two uncles, who lived in Washington State at the time. It felt like I was going back to the second year of school after the school holidays, but instead of school it was back to the army, just it was a different army this time with new basic training, which they call "boot camp". In my head, I thought it was going to be tough, but I never expected it to open my eyes to the extent it did.

I was on the bus going to a three-month Boot Camp at Georgia, Fort Benning, and I will never forget the Sergeant on the bus turning around to me and saying, "Are you ready to wake up at 4am from now on?" I forgot to research that bit, and I thought he was joking, but he wasn't. From that day on, I was up before 5am for the next few years of my life. I couldn't believe it. At this point in my life, The British Army was still the toughest thing I had ever done, but even there we could get away with sleeping in until at least 6am, sometimes until 8am – what a luxury!

During the very first three days, they smoked us (this is a nicer way of saying punished us with physical exercise). It was something I'd never expected. I probably did more push-ups, sit-ups and 'up, down, gos' within those three days than you would think is humanly possible. In those three days, I slept in one room with at least 50 other men, and most of the time we were shoulder to shoulder. We had 4 hours' sleep each night but it was not consecutive – 20 minutes here, an hour there. I didn't speak to another person for three whole days because there was a Drill Sergeant present at all times, who would not allow it. He would not let us rest, day or night.

In the British Army, right from the beginning, we had a little freedom with our nutrition. We had the freedom to walk to the canteen by ourselves, and we had an option to choose what we wanted from the selection available on that day, and we could have as much as we wanted. At night time, if we had any money, we could pop down to the naffy (Army shops) and buy any food/sweets/treats we wanted.

With the US Army, we had no freedom at all with our nutrition. We were marched to the canteen and didn't get to choose what to eat as we went through. They choose for us and would give us one scoop of the thing that they decided we would eat. Then, we had very little time to eat it all. It was a very different experience compared to the British Army.

Before I joined I thought I was mentally and physically tough enough to face anything that came my way, but the US Army opened my eyes more than I could have imagined and made me realise how programmed society is.

Right from the beginning, I was pushed out of my comfort zone and right from the beginning, I had to break the way that I had been programmed in life, even after being in the British Army. I had to be open to new ways of doing things. I had to challenge my personal limitations. I had to change my mindset.

I mean if I told you to wake up at 4am every morning from now you would think that it was abnormal and not right, but when you understand that your life doesn't have to be 9-5, Monday-Friday, the better it can be. I mean if you need something done and it's 9pm, there is nothing stopping you from staying up until midnight and still waking up for work the next day. Yes, you may be tired but you've got it done.

There are 24 hours in the day and I thank the US Army for teaching me how to utilise them.

For the majority of the days, I would be up at 4:30am to start my day. I was fortunate enough to be trained by a special forces soldier, and his mentality was that you cannot go to sleep until your task is done.

While training with the US Army, I gained such an incredible fitness level that I loved everything about fitness. All day every day, I was thinking about what I could do to push myself. It ignited a passion for fitness within me. I remember being in stunning landscapes with beautiful views, and others would admire the view, thinking about the beautiful mountains or countryside. Whereas I would think, 'I wonder if I could run all the way up that mountain without stopping,' or 'I wonder how long it would take me to run up those hills.'

The most rewarding fitness experience I had was when I was in Iraq. One of the soldiers in my platoon had gained a lot of weight and couldn't pass the US Army Physical Fitness Test, which consisted of doing as many push-ups as you can in 2 minutes, as many sit-ups as you can in 2 minutes, and a timed 2-mile run. For the sit-ups and push-ups, there was a minimum requirement you had to meet.

He was so heavy and unfit he was given two weeks to lose weight and pass the test or face disciplinary action. The worst-case scenario was they would ask him to leave the Army.

As I was the one with the biggest passion for fitness within the platoon, he asked for my help. I could feel the pain he was going through and I made it my mission to make sure that he would pass. We put a plan together and for two weeks we had to train before missions, whilst on missions and after missions.

It was a tough two weeks for both of us. Then, the day came when he was to be weighed to make sure he wasn't too heavy to be in the Army, and even though it wouldn't affect my career in any way if he passed or not, I was just as anxious as he was to find out the results. We'd both put so much into it.

I couldn't see him as he was behind a wall, but when I heard him cheer for joy I knew he had passed, which put a big smile on my face. But getting the weight off was the easy part.

Straight after being weighed, the whole platoon had to do the US Army Physical Fitness Test, which meant I could help encourage him with the sit-ups and push-ups, as we were always in view of each other. But when it came to the timed run, he was on his own, as I had to run it at my pace so that I would pass the test. (Humble brag, but that run was the fastest two-miles I have ever run: 11 minutes and 56 seconds.)

Whenever we did the two-mile run, he was always last. However, after two weeks of intense training, I think everyone's jaw hit the floor when they saw him overtaking people who used to be much fitter. Not only that, he also ended up running the 2 miles faster than he had ever done before. This meant he had passed the test, would not be disciplined and was allowed to remain in the Army.

I felt his joy. It was a great feeling for both of us and, from that day on, I knew that one day I wanted to be a personal trainer who helped people to escape a body they felt trapped in.

Throughout our Boot Camp training, we had two drill sergeants assigned to us. One was truly inspirational, and the other wasn't so good. In life, no matter what they are trying to teach you, you have some people who are great at both what they do and how they teach it, and you have others who are great at what they do but prove to be terrible at teaching. This was my experience with the not-so-good drill sergeant, he clearly knew his stuff but the way he taught us was terrible! He should have not been in that position, as he focused more on destroying us than building us up.

The good drill sergeant not only knew his stuff, but he taught it in such a way that it would become ingrained in your head. I still use the things he taught us to this day. He also taught by example. If we had to be up until say 3am, so would he; and if we had to wake up and be ready for 5am, he too would be there with us. He gained everyone's massive respect for what he did for us.

During my time doing British Army Basic Training, I had four sergeants who were assigned to us throughout the 6 months and one captain. Throughout the 6 months, they were incredibly hard on us. Once I was finished with them, I couldn't thank them enough. They were hard and tough on us for the right reasons and helped to build us in the right way.

Having worked under a lot of different 'teachers' in the Army, I knew what it was that made a good and effective one, and that

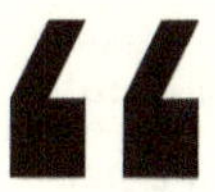

THERE IS NO BETTER FEELING

THAN BEING THE PERSON WHO

IS RESPONSIBLE FOR CHANGING

SOMEONE'S LIFE AND HELPING

THEM TO ESCAPE A BODY THAT

THEY FEEL TRAPPED WITHIN.

was certainly the type of teacher I wanted to be in the next phase of my life.

## BECOMING A PERSONAL TRAINER AND TRAINING SMARTER

Before I became a personal trainer, there were two major events that changed my life. The British Army, which made me barbarically fit, and then the American Army, which opened up my mind and helped me think out of the systematic lifestyle that a lot of people are programmed in.

Whilst in the Army, I found myself becoming a PT to colleagues that needed a bit of help, without ever really intending to. When I left, I decided to commit myself to a life of helping other people to get healthier. However, I was surprised at how little I actually knew regarding health and fitness. Being a personal trainer helped me realise there is so much to learn. Even though I was mentally and physically strong enough to take on any challenge, if I wanted a six-pack, I would have to eat relatively healthily and do a lot of exercise until I had one.

Previously, I thought I had enough knowledge of health and fitness. I was very wrong. Within the first 6 months of becoming a personal trainer, I realised that my fitness levels would have been on another level and, instead of barbarically getting a six-pack, I could have trained so much smarter.

This part of my life made me realise two things: that I should never stop learning and how important integrity is. It is not the end of the world if you do not know something, and admitting this is the best way to try and learn about something.

For example, I know a lot about helping people to escape an unhealthy, overweight body and I can comfortably and confidently help someone to escape, and I still try and learn more about how to do it in better ways.

## TODAY

In my life, I have helped to build houses and buildings. I have been in two different armies. I have been to war for 12 months and completed over 300 combat missions. (Just to clarify this, one combat mission could be something very simple, such as driving the colonel to meet with an Iraqi official for breakfast.) But there is no better feeling than being the person who is responsible for changing someone's life and helping them to escape a body that they feel trapped within and live a life they can only dream of.

When I was growing up, I never felt free and was stuck in a body that I despised. I was always afraid to take on any physical challenges or life challenges because I didn't believe in myself and I had no pride. Now I crave finding people who want and need to break free.

If this is YOU, from today, grab life by the horns and take control, so you can gain the **FREEDOM** to enjoy the life you desire and feel comfortable enough within your body to wear what you want, when you want. I want to give you the confidence and happiness that comes with feeling healthy. I want you to be **FEARLESS** towards life's challenges that come your way, both mentally and physically. And I want you to do it all with **PRIDE.** Just like I have done during my life and career.

# PART 1

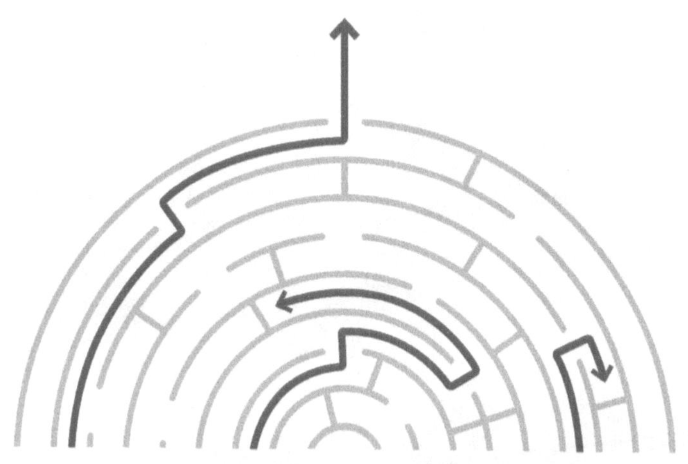

# GET YOUR OBSTACLES
# OUT THE WAY

# INTRODUCTION TO PART 1

This time is going to be different. I know you may have tried all sorts of exercise and diet plans before but what I do differently is identify what level you are at and then work out what's right for you. You wouldn't get someone who can barely walk to the shops to enter a marathon straight away, and it's the same with nutrition. It's about building up from where you are now to where you want to be in a slow, manageable and sustainable way.

But before we dive in, it is important you understand three things, which I will explore in-depth in part 1. These are:

1. Emotions and hormones

2. Bad habits

3. Knowledge

To put it simply, if you do not understand these three things they will control you and your body. Once you understand them you have a much better chance of being in control of your body.

**Emotions and hormones** are suppressed with **bad habits.** This is because you do not have the **knowledge** to know how to suppress them in a healthier and better way.

Emotions and hormones play a very big role in losing weight because they create bad habits. The longer you feed your emotions and hormones with bad habits the harder it is to reverse.

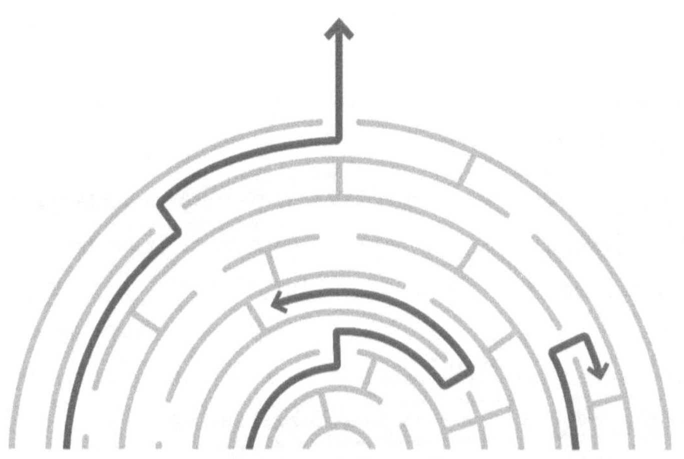

# OBSTACLE 1
## Emotions and Hormones

### WHAT ARE HORMONES?

Hormones are chemical messengers that transport signals from one cell to another and play a vital role when you're trying to lose weight.

- **Cortisol** is known as the stress hormone. The more cortisol that your body creates the more stress you may feel.

- **Dopamine** is thought of as a "happy hormone". The more of it your body creates, the happier you feel.

- **Insulin** is a hormone that allows your body to use sugar (glucose) from the foods you eat for energy or to store glucose for future use.

## How your emotion and hormones can create habits

When people have high cortisol levels, they experience the emotion of stress. Often, they will try to counteract it by eating sugary treats, like a slice of cake or chocolate, which will trigger dopamine and give them a feel-good boost. However, this sugar will then spike their insulin levels, which gives them a ton of energy for a period of time. Then, after a while, their energy levels drop and, because they lack energy, they reach for something sugary to boost them up again and the cycle repeats itself.

Let's say you have created a bad habit and now every time you get stressed you eat something sweet like chocolate to give you a feel-good boost. Then, one day, you decide not to eat chocolate when you feel stressed. What can actually happen is that you will feel even more stressed than usual because your body is so used to having sugar when it is stressed, and your body gets confused as to why you are not doing what you normally do, and so craves the chocolate. However, don't let this put you off, because your body will adapt after a while, just remember that when you next start a new diet.

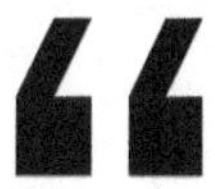

I AM NOT SAYING YOU SHOULDN'T

EVER HAVE ANYTHING SWEET.

WHAT I AM SAYING IS TRY AND

LEARN TO HAVE A TREAT FOR

WHEN IT IS ACTUALLY A TREAT

THAT YOU WILL ENJOY, NOT JUST

TO COVER UP AN EMOTION.

The higher your insulin and cortisol levels are, the harder it is to lose weight.

Now, I am not saying you shouldn't ever have anything sweet. What I am saying is try and learn to have a treat for when it is actually a treat that you will enjoy, not just to cover up an emotion. You need to learn to release different emotions with good habits.

For example, if you are stressed and you want a feel-good boost from dopamine, instead of eating something sugary, going for a walk will also boost your dopamine levels. It is far healthier and the dopamine good feeling will last longer.

When you have created a habit, your hormones and body will be used to it, and so when you try to change it for a healthier habit, your hormones may fight against that change, which results in cravings until your body has adapted to this and breaks the craving.

For example, if you created a habit of drinking a cup of unhealthy hot chocolate every night before going to bed and you try to stop it in order to be healthier, your hormones will create emotions at first that will make you desperately want a cup. Then you will end up having a debate inside your head as to why you should have a cup of hot chocolate. One voice will tell you why you should have the hot chocolate, and the other will tell you why you shouldn't. If you don't have a strong mindset, your emotions will overpower you and the voice telling you to have the hot chocolate will win. However, you must persist in trying to break the hot chocolate habit because it can take up to three months before you completely stop craving it, but if you persist, your body adapts and you will break the habit for good.

One of my most favourite sayings is by Mike Tyson, who learnt it from his trainer: "I have the discipline to do the things I hate, but I will do it like I love it."

You can actually set your mind to do this when your body and emotions and hormones are not agreeing with you. I used to do this in the Army. There were a lot of times when we were in situations where we were not able to eat as much as we needed, and we would be very hungry. I remember feeling so hungry it felt slightly painful, and when it kicked in, I used to tell myself that it was a sign of accomplishment. Then I started to enjoy that feeling when I felt it.

## WHY ARE HORMONES IMPORTANT?

Hormones are like an orchestra. When everyone in an orchestra is playing in tune, the music sounds wonderful and creates great emotions for the audience. But if one musical instrument is off, the whole performance is off. It's the same with your body; if just one hormone is not in balance, it will create havoc in your body.

The great news is you are the conductor. You largely control how your body is being played because you decide what you put inside your body, and what you do with your body will determine the outcome.

You will achieve a much better outcome if you do a minimum of 30 minutes of exercise and fill yourself with good nutrition each day, rather than sitting around, not doing any activity and filling yourself up with processed food daily.

## HOW DO HORMONES AFFECT EMOTIONS?

When our hormones are imbalanced, they can trigger negative emotions, such as anxiety, low mood and the feeling that you don't want to do anything. We need to be careful how we respond to emotions because if we're not attentive, we can make that hormone imbalance even greater and end up feeling worse.

For example, and you might be able to relate to this, some people try to suppress the stress they feel with bad habits, like unhealthy comfort food or a few glasses of wine (or maybe even both). If your bad habit is unhealthy food, the instant gratification feels great but the after-effects which normally start straight away will leave you feeling sluggish, demotivated, tired and unhappy. If you keep repeating this every time you are stressed it obviously creates a bad outcome. Your stress hormone (cortisol) will run riot and your insulin levels will be high as your body tries to process all the sugars you've consumed and your happy hormone has a day off.

The good thing is we can flip this. Some people who feel stressed will suppress this emotion with good habits, like exercise or doing rewarding things. This might be going for a walk, taking 5 minutes' quiet time for themselves or having a relaxing bath. With all of these things, there may be gratification, but it won't be instant because the stress hormone will reduce and the happiness hormone will increase. In the long term, however, these activities help to keep your happy hormone levels healthy, leaving you less open to attack from the stress hormone.

This is very important to understand when you try to escape an unhealthy, overweight body.

## ALCOHOL: THE QUICKEST WAY TO MESS UP YOUR HORMONAL AND EMOTIONAL BALANCE

Drinking alcohol will prevent you from losing weight and is a depressant, so it obviously affects your mood. Every time you drink a glass of wine you are pretty much drinking a glass of depressant. Now, you may be thinking, no, it makes me feel happy and relaxed. Yes, but that's only because it gives you instant gratification, but the after-effect is dangerous. Let me explain how it affected me so badly.

# MY STORY: EMOTIONAL DEPENDENCE ON ALCOHOL

I was a binge drinker, so I would drink all weekend if I could get away with it. I always knew it wasn't very good for me but I didn't realise how bad it was until I completely stopped.

I always had patches when I would stop drinking for a month. When I did stop drinking for a month or so my life would be so much better, but then I would remember how much fun it was and very quickly lose my motivation and end up back to drinking every weekend. And that is when the trouble would start again.

If I was to drink on a Saturday night, I would have the instant gratification it provided but I would wake up on Sunday with a terrible hangover, feeling really down and focussing on all the negative things in my life. On Monday, I would just feel tired and slightly hungover and miserable, but by Tuesday I thought I was over it. I wouldn't feel ill and I would have energy, but mentally I felt depressed.

This is the dangerous part; I didn't know that my sadness half-way through the week was caused by my drinking on Saturday night. And every time you drink, your depression and all the other bad feelings you have will accumulate.

One Christmas, I had enough of feeling crap and I decided I was going to stop drinking for 1 year. When I first tried to stop my binge drinking, my body expected alcohol at the weekend.

It was ready and expecting it, but didn't get any. This created anxiety as my body could not understand why the pattern had been broken and it wasn't having alcohol anymore. Then the hormones in my body would create strong emotional feelings to try and get me back to my usual drinking routine, as my body was dependent on alcohol and preparing for it. It had become the expected norm, and my body didn't like changing the pattern. It took 3 months for the cravings to stop, and only then could I start to feel the real benefits of being sober. This created an indescribable wave of emotions that made me feel happy on a level I cannot describe.

This relates to every bad habit. If you are used to eating chocolate three times a day or having a glass of wine straight after work every night, or doing something that you know is affecting your ability to lose weight, your body will need chocolate or wine or that craving every day to feel normal.

After 5 months of not drinking, I started to realise why I drank so much. Again, you may be able to relate to this. I found out I wasn't drinking to have fun, but to escape a life I felt trapped in. When you get drunk, it helps you forget about everything that has happened in the past or may in the future. For the 4-8 hours you are out drinking and partying, you focus on the present of the night, but as soon as the next day arrives and you are no longer drinking, reality hits and then you realise, you still have bills to pay, but now with less money or you are still unhealthy. Added to that, you're no closer to escaping your body and developing the one you desire, or you are still

“

THE WORSE THE WEIGHT
PROBLEM, THE WORSE THE
MENTAL HEALTH PROBLEM.

”

depressed but now even more depressed because you spent all night long drinking depressants (alcohol). The effect that alcohol has on your mentality is extremely dangerous.

Once I'd stopped, I had more time to spend on the other problems that were keeping me from the left side of the happy scale and I became consciously aware of what I needed to do to get over to the right side.

It is a hard and horrible emotional journey trying to break habits and everyone around you will suffer at first because you can become very short-tempered as you experience the emotional and hormonal imbalances. You won't be able to function properly and everyone will annoy you more than usual. Just remember, the longer you take to break the habit the harder it is.

Although my own story is about being emotionally dependent on alcohol, you may be emotionally dependent on something else – maybe you comfort eat or have other vices or addictions that are distracting you from being happy, healthy and confident.

Figure them out and crush them.

## WEIGHT AND MENTAL HEALTH

The longer you carry your weight (fat), the greater the effect it is going to have, not only on your body but also on your emotions and hormones.

The worse the weight problem, the worse the mental health problem.

Let me put this in a way that you might understand better. Soldiers increase their fitness through numerous methods. One of them is to carry a burgeon (rucksack) for miles on end that is sometimes twice their own body weight.

Throughout this carry (fitness session) there will be a point where a soldier thinks about breaking his/her own leg, just so he/she can get out of having to carry it any further. I can vouch for this. I contemplated it many times.

When it comes to carrying weight, including your body weight, you will only be able to carry it around for so long. After that, you are going to think of extreme ways to get out of your pain and misery. In some sad cases, people's mental health can deteriorate to the point they become desperate and suicidal. Don't let that happen.

## COMPARISON IS THE THIEF OF HAPPINESS

Another one of my favourite quotes is, 'Comparison is the thief of happiness.'

The only person you should be competing against in this journey is yourself; you will let in a lot of negative emotions if you start comparing yourself to others.

By all means, have friendly competitions with people who are on the same journey as you, as these will help you stay focused, but don't start comparing your body or achievement to someone else's.

I used to weigh and measure my clients with a tape that would tell me how many inches they had on different parts of their body so they could keep track of their journeys, but on numerous occasions, people would be disheartened with their results because someone else had done better.

People, on average, lose 14lb (6kg) and 2 clothes sizes (dress or trouser sizes) within the first month with me.

This one time, I had a lady who lost 14lb and 2 dress sizes but because someone else had lost 21lb she felt that she hadn't achieved anything, and did not celebrate losing a whole 14lb because of this comparison. I explained how well she had done but she still wasn't happy because someone else had done better.

This has happened a number of times, which blows my mind. Even after I have explained how well they have done they are still unhappy because they are comparing themselves with someone else.

In this journey, it is you, the mirror and your mind.

# MY STORY: CONTROL YOUR EMOTIONS OR YOUR EMOTIONS WILL CONTROL YOU

You have to control your emotions because if you don't, bad consequences can happen.

In 2010, I went to Kirkuk in Iraq with the US Army on an operation called Operation New Dawn. I was a part of a team called PSD (personal security detail) for the Colonel and Sergeant Major.

Whenever the base was attacked, a different kind of alarm would go off, with each one indicating what kind of attack it was.

I will never forget how one day, my friend Ramon (the driver of the Humvee I was in) and I were dismantling the equipment from the Humvee. The base alarm went off (which indicated that something was being fired at the base – normally a mortar). When this alarm goes off, you should just seek cover. The safest places on the base were these little makeshift bunkers that were dotted around. However, my friend and I were quite far away from a bunker. So, we calmly took a seat in the Humvee because it had a level of protection.

As we looked through the window of the Humvee, it was like watching a dark comedy sketch. In the distance, the base postman was running as fast as he could (while still holding on to his parcels) into a bunker. He should have just got underneath the armoured vehicle that he was standing by.

One of the other men from my platoon (Ramol) was just looking up into the sky trying to find the mortar, as if he was searching for a shooting star. Then my roommate casually walked past the front of the Humvee repeating, 'Please land on me.' This is a true story.

When the alarm rang, people panicked or acted in unhelpful ways because their emotions were controlling their actions and putting them at risk.

No matter what the scenario, your emotions determine your outcome and this is where knowledge plays a part. Being in an unhealthy, overweight body is a dangerous situation to be in, your health is at risk every day.

When the alarms we had on the base rang, we had to make quick smart decisions to make sure we stayed safe, just like you do if you want to escape an unhealthy, overweight body. Every day, on your journey to escaping an unhealthy, overweight body, you are going to have to make tough decisions.

You can be like the base postman and panic and run to the first weight-loss programme you see or hear about because you don't know any better. If you do, you will be questioning each step you take every day and wondering if it will work or not.

IN THIS JOURNEY, IT IS YOU,

THE MIRROR AND YOUR MIND.

Or you can be like Ramon and me. Take the time to learn what you need to do and understand it's going to be a long journey, be calm along the way and take the right actions with the least risk to your health.

You can be like Ramol and think it is funny, and not give a crap about your health until it hits you in the face with life-threatening conditions. Ramol was just stupid... Do not be like Ramol.

Or you can be like my roommate and just give up on life.

Your life is in your hands, and so are the outcomes of your emotions and hormones.

## • HORMONES AND EMOTIONS TASK •

This is an awareness task that I call **100 emotions**.

This can work in a lot of different ways, but for now, we are going to try and identify which of your emotions trigger bad nutritional habits.

### Step 1

Print a sheet off with this table (which you can download for free on my website: **www.chrismarcoflores.com**) that is set out like this, or draw your own on a blank sheet of paper. You will need 3 columns:

| Time | Consumption (food and fluid intake) | Emotion |
| --- | --- | --- |
|  |  |  |
|  |  |  |

## Step 2

For the next 7 days, every time you eat or drink anything (water doesn't count) fill this out. Like this.

| Time | Consumption (food and fluid intake) | Emotion |
| --- | --- | --- |
| 06:30am | Coffee and toast with butter and jam | Tired, weak & fed-up |
| 6pm | Pizza and wine | Relaxed & exhausted |

## Step 3

Now you can rearrange your table into four buckets like this. The best way to do this is to highlight each bucket with a different colour highlighter.

*Bucket 1* – Sugary treats or caffeine – biscuits/cookies, energy drinks, coffee/tea, cakes

*Bucket 2* – Alcohol

*Bucket 3* – Processed food – unhealthy takeaways (pizza, McDonald's, Chinese etc.)

*Bucket 4* – Other

## Step 4

You will then be able to identify which emotions and times of the day are triggering your bad nutritional habits.

## Step 5

Try to change one bad habit at a time and spend 1 month changing one single bad habit for a good habit. (If you can do more than one at a time then by all means do, but I suggest you start slowly.) Once you have changed one habit, move on to the next.

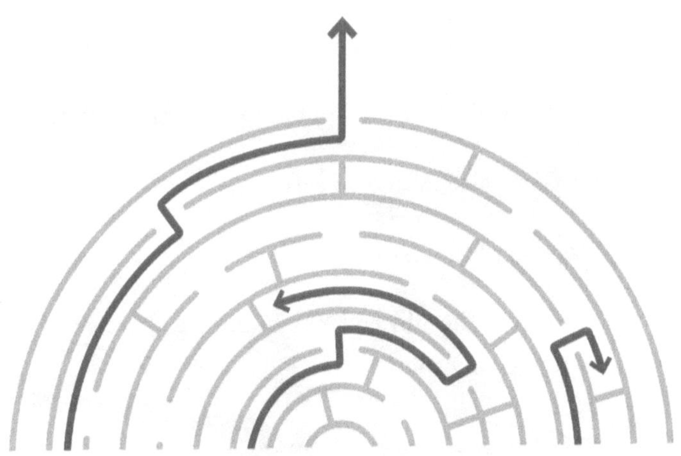

# CHAPTER 2

# OBSTACLE 2
# Bad habits

## WHAT ARE BAD HABITS?

The definition of a bad habit is: a negative behaviour pattern. Habits are patterns of behaviour that you may or may not be aware of. These are patterns that you may have built up over time without realising. People who are successful have a lot of good habits, people who are unsuccessful have a lot of bad habits. You have more habits than you could imagine.

**You may not realise it but your habits will determine what you do achieve or don't achieve in life.**

People who are overweight, unfit and unhealthy tend to have these four common bad habits:

- Don't exercise

- Eat processed foods and unhealthy snacks regularly

- Consume alcohol and/or party regularly

- Have very little sleep

People who are fit, healthy and look healthy tend to have these four common good habits:

- Exercise regularly

- Consume healthy food and drinks

- Drink a lot of water

- Have an adequate amount of sleep

People who have more of these good habits can get away with having processed food or a night out every now and then because their good habits far outweigh their bad ones.

# WHY ARE BAD HABITS IMPORTANT?

Bad habits are what I call "creepers". People who are overweight don't wake up one day and want to be overweight, it happens when lots of little bad habits creep in over time. They repeat the same thing over and over again until it becomes a necessity in their life.

Let me show you a good example of how a bad habit can be built. Imagine if everyone was talking about the TV series *Friends*. You never watch it, and people keep talking about it so much that you want to see what it's all about. So one night you sit down and watch the first two episodes. From that moment on, you are hooked and love the show so much you can't get enough of it.

Then, every night after you finish work, just before you go to bed you watch two or three episodes. Just note, there are 236 episodes and it would probably take you 3 months to watch them all at this rate.

So, now you have created a habit by unwinding every night by watching *Friends*, not only that but you have also started to eat half a packet of biscuits and drink a glass of milk whilst you are watching every night, and this continues for the whole 3 months until it has finished.

After three months, you have created a habit of "unwinding" and comforting yourself by watching two or three episodes and eating half a packet of biscuits before you go to bed.

Now, the TV series of *Friends* may be finished but your craving and bad habit of eating half a packet of biscuits every night before you go to bed will remain. The problem won't just be the bad habit of eating biscuits, it will be the sugar tolerance you will have built up. Your body will now crave more and more sugar around that time of night. This will not help you sleep well.

## LET'S LOOK AT SOME DAILY HABITS

Your morning routine is most likely to be the same. You may be the sort of person who wakes up and gets out of bed before the alarm or hits the snooze button right until the last second you have to get out of bed. Some people will brush their teeth then eat breakfast, others eat breakfast and then brush their teeth. Some people don't even eat breakfast, they just wash, and some don't do that either! If that is you, it's highly recommended that you wash in the morning :)

If you go to work every morning, there are most likely multiple ways that you can get there and you probably use the same route the majority of the time out of habit.

When you get to work, you will most likely do the same things; if you are an office worker, the first thing you might do is put the kettle on and have a coffee in the same mug every day.

When it comes to lunchtime, you go to the same places. (Notice how I said same places. Not place.) Now let's say you go to Nando's, you probably have the same meal each time (I

"

WHEN YOU CONSCIOUSLY

UNDERSTAND THE THINGS THAT

ARE HABITS IN YOUR LIFE, YOU CAN

START BREAKING THEM.

"

know because I do, and I very rarely change), which is a habit I have created.

These habits go on throughout the whole day until you come home. You may be someone who goes to sleep by reading a book on a certain side of the bed or watches TV programmes or a film on the same side of the sofa. These are all habits.

The great thing with habits is you can break them and the more you understand about breaking habits the easier it is to break the harder ones. Let's start by breaking some easier habits. Try going to work a different way every morning, using a different cup every time you have a coffee, reading your book in a different place (not in your bed), and ordering something different for lunch.

When you consciously understand the things that are habits in your life, you can start breaking them.

If you are someone who is on a weight-loss journey then it is important to build your willpower up to the point that you are able to break habits, because when you try to lose weight, I guarantee there are a lot of bad habits to reduce. For example, if you have too much unhealthy chocolate than you will have to reduce the amount of chocolate that you eat.

Go on, be a rebel, go start breaking habits!

# MY STORY: DITCHING THE ALARM CLOCK

This is another life lesson I learned while I was in Kirkuk, Iraq.

We carried out a combat mission nearly every day for the whole 12 months we were there. Sometimes we did 2 missions in one day. You are probably thinking: my God, this boy has seen some action. This is not the case. Some missions would consist of escorting the Colonel from our camp to go a police compound to see a Middle-Eastern Commander for breakfast where they would discuss war tactics or the latest episode of *Friends*! Then other missions were extremely serious, as you can imagine.

The majority of our days would be different. Some days we would have to be ready to go at 4am and others we wouldn't have to leave until 12pm, so our body clocks were all over the place.

I created a habit of doing without an alarm. No matter what time I needed to wake up, I would not set an alarm clock. If I needed to be up at 3am, I would wake up before 3am and start the day as normal. It's an extreme example of how a habit is broken.

You probably think that is impossible, but imagine if alarms had never been invented and you had to rely on yourself to wake up. Would you not wake up or would you learn to wake up when needed?

## BAD FOOD HABITS AND THE SCIENCE OF WEIGHT LOSS

To lose weight and get into great shape, you have to change your bad eating habits.

Before I go into this, let me briefly give you a little science on how to lose weight. You need a certain number of calories a day to maintain your body weight. Let's say you need 2500 calories to maintain your weight. If you consume more than this (e.g. 3000 calories) you will put on weight and if you consume less than this (e.g. 1500 calories) you will lose weight. Therefore, if you need 2500 calories a day, you can have 1500 calories of cheesecake and lose weight or 1500 calories of lean chicken and vegetables and lose weight. It is as simple as that.

Or is it? The more muscle you have on your body, the quicker you will burn fat. Protein feeds your muscles and helps them to continue to develop, along with other macro and micronutrients (carbs, fats, vitamins and minerals). Your body is going to utilise a meal of chicken and vegetables a lot more than it will cheesecake, because it provides your body with a lot more nutrients.

If you eat nothing but processed foods, pizza, takeaways, burgers, cakes and sweets, and only hydrate with sugary drinks or alcohol every day, you are not going to lose weight. This MUST change. I'm not saying you have to completely cut out all the most delicious foods and treats, but you are going to have to cut right down, forever!

You have to break the habits. If you like drinking Coke every single day, the sugar will be the main thing you crave and then the flavour. In fact, if you went into a restaurant and they didn't have any Coke, I'll bet my bottom dollar you will still have a fizzy drink. It'll just be a different flavour, like a Sprite. The sugar and chemicals in the Sprite will satisfy your needs, and if you drink enough Sprite over a period of time, your body is going to crave it regularly.

## BAD FOOD HABITS VS GOOD FOOD HABITS

Let me explain the outcomes of eating something bad vs eating something good.

**Eating badly:** You know the feeling when you really want something bad, like a kebab, Chinese or McDonald's, and your eyes are bigger than your belly.

As you eat it, you start to feel satisfied because of the delicious taste, but near enough instantly afterwards you feel physically sick and then about 10 minutes after that you feel tired and sluggish. About 40 minutes later, you start to feel sad and the next day you have a food hangover feeling or become depressed. This is the fault of the poor nutritional choice you made, and it's affecting all your hormones, which are now playing like a really bad orchestra.

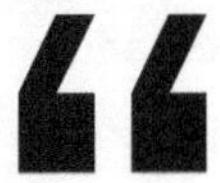

SUBSTITUTING YOUR BAD
HABITS FOR SIMILAR THINGS IS
THE DEVIL'S SECOND FAVOURITE
TOOL TO PREVENT YOU FROM
CHANGING. (THE FIRST TOOL
IS ALCOHOL.)

Your nutrition is a big contributing factor if you have any of the following: insomnia, depression, anxiety, poor health, poor physical abilities.

**Eating well:** Now imagine you changed that meal and pigged out on, say, a healthy BBQ of grilled lean meat/fish with a big green salad and a lot of fresh water. You may need to sit down straight away to let your food go down, but not long after you will be full of energy, feel happy and be ready to get active. You'll also end up having a good night's sleep and the next day you will be raring to go. This is because you have fed your body with good nutrition, which it can utilise throughout your body to benefit it in every way.

Having something as little as a chocolate bar can knock you off your stride, affect your focus and make you feel sluggish, tired, stressed and slightly depressed. Changing that chocolate bar for a handful of nuts will make a great difference.

## WHAT HAVE YOU GOT YOUR BODY USED TO?

Do you ever find that it is so easy to put weight on and it would be easier to get an elephant to breakdance than to get that weight off again?

I will tell you why that is right now. Let's say hypothetically you are 280lb (127kg) and have been for a few years. This means your body's standard set weight is 280lb. When you lose weight and drop to 266lb (121kg), your body starts to create havoc because it's not at its comfortable set weight, which is 280lb. Your body will then do everything it can to get you back to what it is used to.

Your temptations will increase and your subconscious mind will start playing tricks by asking you why you are bothering to lose weight and questioning whether it's all worth it. As a result, you will notice food 100 times more than normal.

Your hormones, once again, play a big part in this, especially in the stomach. Every time you eat, it sends a message to your brain telling you that you're eating. Now say, if you eat 100 times a day, that would be 100 messages sent to your brain (we could take this one step further by adding the amount you eat as well, but let's keep it simple). If you went from eating 100 times a day to eating only 50 times a day, your brain is going to be signalling saying, 'why are you not eating?' Again, this sends your body into havoc because it doesn't understand why you are changing.

Trying to reset your set weight is extremely difficult, and if you do not break the back of this task you will end up back at that weight. Being half into a diet and half out is not setting yourself up to win.

Losing weight and putting it back on is a long-term habit or pattern and if you do not focus on changing your lifestyle by changing your habits, you could end up trying to lose weight for the rest of your life.

## BE CAREFUL ABOUT SWAPPING ONE BAD HABIT FOR ANOTHER

Substituting your bad habits for similar things is the devil's second favourite tool to prevent you from changing. (The first tool is alcohol.)

Imagine that you drink a lot of Coke, so much that it's the main reason you cannot lose weight. Imagine that you've been drinking 10 cans of Coke a day, but you start to substitute this for 10 cans of Diet Coke because it has little to no calories. Do you think that's a healthy choice? In this scenario, you're not teaching your body to break the habit, only to substitute it. If you satisfy your body with a similar product, it will only be a matter of time before you go back to the original product. 'Out of sight out of mind.' Break the habit and you will break the temptation.

In my experience, the clients I have trained who only substitute habits for similar habits instead of cutting the habit out altogether, struggle to lose any weight because their body is still craving that particular habit.

Clients who focus on breaking the habits and cutting out all the stuff that prevents them from losing weight not only get the best results, but also feel fantastic, look the greatest and continue to get results after they have finished with me.

Imagine if a doctor told you that if you drank one more can of Coke you would drop dead! I'm pretty sure you would probably never drink a can of Coke again. That is an extreme example.

You can start by only having Coke on just two days a week, but it has to be two different days each week. If you get used to having your treat on a Saturday, you will look forward to that treat every Saturday. However, if you swap the days around every week then you will disrupt and weaken your habits, which makes them easier to break.

## CASE STUDY: SARA

*Sara became a client and a very close friend very quickly. I first met Sara in October 2017 when she was 54 years old. Sara weighed 227lbs (103kg) stood at 5ft. 3inches and she told me when we first met that she had been on many diets and would lose lots of weight (up to 70lbs/31kg) and then put it all back on.*

*Then she would pick another diet and repeat the process, and this went on for 10 years. Sara had had enough. She had pre-paid for a gastric band, which I personally feel is an awful way to lose weight, but came to see me before she did it. We had a long conversation during which I encouraged her to concentrate on changing her lifestyle.*

*Sara's nemesis was alcohol. She would drink wine every weekday. Then at the weekend, she and her friends would drink until they couldn't walk, and this had been her life for years! When I told her that I would only allow her to come on my course if she stopped drinking alcohol, it was a huge shock because she couldn't imagine life without drinking. It was a key factor as to whether she was going to sign up with me or not.*

*To convince her, I used a tactic that people may disagree with, but I don't care because it works incredibly well. It's called 'dig for pain'. A lot of people only change when they are in real pain and sometimes wait until they hit life-threatening situations before they do – like being diagnosed with diabetes, or being told their blood pressure is so high they can't even have an operation. My technique is to be truthful as it helps clients to open up their eyes and mind to see what will happen if they do not change. It could be an early death or not being able to enjoy their kids or grandkids the way they'd like to in the future because they will be so restricted with their physical abilities.*

*I knew Sara was desperate to lose weight, so I asked a series of questions to make her realise how serious her situation was (which I will put up in the mindset section). It was an emotional session, but it really helped her to dig deep down. It shook her up enough to understand that she had to change. Sara didn't want to cancel her gastric band because she wasn't sure that my plan would work. I asked her to give me 12 weeks before going down that route.*

*Sara agreed to join me and not drink any alcohol for a minimum of three months. I knew she wouldn't last three months without drinking any alcohol, but the idea was to change her mindset and make her so determined she would even give up the thing that gave her the most comfort in life. The day we had that conversation, she went from drinking every day to not drinking a single drop for 2 weeks.*

*When she did drink, Sara felt guilty and told me straight away (which was great because I knew she wouldn't last and telling me showed me how serious she was and how much she was trying). After that blip, she didn't drink anything else for the rest of the time, and as a result, I received a text 6 weeks later saying she had cancelled her gastric band. Just 12 weeks later, Sara had lost 4 dress sizes and dropped 42lbs (19kg). That is the power of the mind.*

*If you are in so much pain that you want to change, your number one priority is getting yourself into a healthy mindset. Stop looking for the next holiday, new car, or night out. Before making every decision just ask yourself this question: Is this going to help me with my weight loss or affect it? Do the right thing.*

**'Treat the mind as a muscle, the more you train it, the stronger it becomes.'**

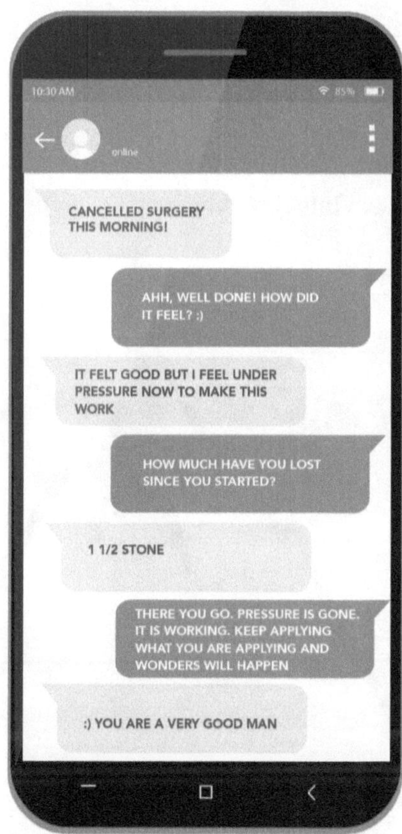


SURGERY CANCELLED!

# THE MOUNTAIN ANALOGY

When you climb a mountain, you have to climb to the top and then once you reach the summit, you have to climb down. If you have never climbed a mountain, then let me tell you that physically, climbing down can be just as hard as climbing up, but mentally, coming down is a lot easier, because the end goal is in sight.

I want you to imagine every time you start a new diet that you are at the bottom of the mountain and every time you lose weight you get closer to the top. The higher you go the harder it becomes, just like climbing a mountain and burning fat. Let's split this mountain into three horizontal sections.

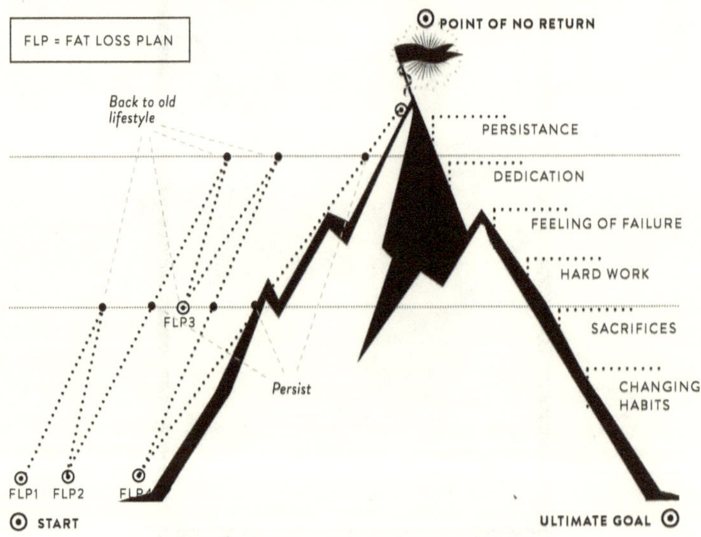


CONQUERING THE MOUNTAIN

Most people do not get past the first section because it not only gets harder, but they also feel like they have achieved enough already and stop trying to achieve any more. These people end up going back down to the bottom of the mountain and having to start again. Some people make it into the second section and stop when they get to the third, and only a handful ever make it past the third section and to the top.

If you break through the sections and persist to the top of the mountain, you will hit the point of no return, because you have to get down one way or another. The top of the mountain is not your end goal. Oh no! You still have to come down the mountain, but you have done the hard part and mentally it's nearly over.

Your weight-loss journey is the same. As people start losing weight and are just about to go into the second or third section, they feel like they have lost enough weight. They feel better and look better, so they treat themselves more often and start going back to their old lifestyle. Before they know it, they have put all their weight back on and are back to square one at the bottom of the mountain. And then, after a while, they seek another diet (mountain) to tackle because they have convinced themselves the last one didn't work when, in fact, they just didn't stick to it. Can you relate to this? It is called yoyo dieting.

Stop chasing diets. Let me ask you a question. How many diets have you been on in your life to try and lose weight? If your answer is a lot, then you need to stop chasing the next diet. The problem with us humans is we always want the next thing or new things.

Like a car, for example. If you brought the latest BMW it will be the coolest thing ever! However, this same car will look old in 20 years' time and you will want to upgrade to a newer model. Yet, it is still running and can do the same thing. Well, that is what you are doing with these diets, always looking for the one everyone is talking about. Then, once you have tried it, and found out that it does not work as well as you'd hoped, it becomes a useless diet.

You may have to adapt diets along the way as you improve, which is another story. The most important thing is to stop letting your excuses get in the way, such as I have to drink this weekend it's my sister's wedding or it's my son's birthday and I will have to eat cake to celebrate with him.

If you persist on your journey to the top of the mountain, you will hit the point of no return and have the greatest feeling in the world. You will feel invincible, like you can take on any challenge. You will look at yourself and know that you may need to lose more weight or get into better shape, but you will feel fearless because you know you can do it. By this time, you will have created good healthy habits, so making good choices no longer feels like a chore. You will also have become one of those people who you may find annoying because they post about going to the gym 7 times a day and how they're looking forward to their avocado and kale smoothie. (You may be reading this and thinking that will never happen to you; get to the top of that mountain and see for yourself.)

How do you know when you are at the top of the mountain? I'm guessing you brush your teeth every day. Okay, if that is a yes then, no matter how late you wake up and how busy your day ahead of you is, you will find a way to brush your teeth.

When you get to a level of fitness and health, your body craves fitness and health. If you do not exercise one day, you will feel as out of sorts as you do when you don't brush your teeth. When you get yourself used to a level of health and love feeling healthy, you can be in a room full of takeaways and not have the urge to eat anything bad. That is when you know you have hit the top of the mountain.

If you have never experienced that feeling of being on top of a mountain, it's hard to understand what it's like, and I encourage you to seek that experience, even if it is just once in your life. It's the greatest feeling in the world.

One of the best ways to start climbing the mountain is to identify your bad habits (which you did in the emotion and hormones task on page 61) and take the time to break them one by one (or two by two if you have a strong enough mindset) and then replace each bad habit with a good one.

## • BREAK THE HABIT TASK •

Remember, the more you train your brain the stronger it gets as you can learn to break habits every day, with little actions.

This task aims to consciously break your habits and to strengthen your WILLpower.

If you have done the previous challenge on page 61, 'Emotion and hormone task', this will help you to complete this task.

### Step 1

Look at the table and pick one thing off it that is clearly a bad habit, which you consume daily (if you didn't fill in the table, think of something you crave which you know is not good for you).

## Step 2

Tempt yourself with this particular habit and consciously change it for a good healthy habit. For example, if your bad habit is a chocolate bar every lunchtime, then I want you to get one at lunchtime, open it and put it in front of you. You can then either chuck it in the bin or give it to someone else and consume something healthy instead, like a handful of nuts or fruit.

## Step 3

Do this for 10 days and then after that time, don't tempt yourself with the bad, just go straight for the good.

## Step 4

Do this with a new habit every month until you have got rid of all your bad habits and they have turned into good ones.

At first, you are not going to feel satisfied, but you will feel like you have accomplished something. It will be easier to turn away other "bad" things in future because you have prepared your body to do so.

> YOU SHOULD THINK OF YOUR BODY
> AND HEALTH IN THE SAME WAY
> THAT ATHLETES THINK OF THE
> OLYMPICS. AN ATHLETE'S REWARD
> FOR WINNING THE OLYMPICS
> IS A GOLD MEDAL. HOWEVER,
> YOUR GOLD MEDAL IS BEING AT A
> HEALTHY AND FIT LEVEL.

# HABITS AND CONSISTENCY

You don't see a gold medallist turn up at the Olympics and just expect a gold medal! No. They train extremely hard for years in advance until they are ready to win. Then, once they have got their gold medal, they can relax (unless they are training for another one). However, they will still maintain their fitness and health and can be seen exercising and eating healthy regularly.

I cannot stress how important consistency is. When you embark on a journey that is going to help you escape an unhealthy, over-weight body, you must understand that if you want long-lasting results, you are going to have to do it for the rest of your life. I'm talking about long-term habits here.

For example, if you are overweight and you sign up to a 3-month weight-loss course, you shouldn't go into it thinking that you are going to do this for 3 months and then you can relax. You must go into it thinking, I am now going to implement what they teach me for the rest of my life.

The quicker you increase your health and fitness levels, the quicker you will enjoy it and the quicker it will become a part of your life. Whereas, the longer you leave it, the harder it will be to make it a part of your life.

You should think of your body and health in the same way that athletes think of the Olympics. An athlete's reward for winning the Olympics is a gold medal. However, your gold medal is being at a healthy and fit level. You should be doing something every single day to achieve that gold medal.

# CASE STUDY: CLAIRE

*Before coming to me, Claire trained for 4 years and didn't lose much weight. She dropped 42lbs (19kg) in 12 weeks with me, however. When she first met me, she was a size 22, had tried a lot of diets and had exercised regularly for the past 4 years.*

*She would always lose a bit of weight, and then put it back on. That happened for 4 years. Claire was confused. She felt she was doing all the right things and didn't understand why she wasn't losing the weight.*

*So, I drilled down and found out what she was doing wrong. She was doing the right thing with exercising but not with the intensity that was needed.*

*She was eating well but a few things were holding her back (the little treats and the small amount of alcohol that she had at night to keep her happy). But these little things were throwing her hormones out of balance, which prevented her weight loss.*

*By tweaking a few little things, putting her through the levels of nutrition and increasing her exercise intensity levels and making her 'fear the sessions' (which you will under-stand later in this book), she dropped 4 dress sizes, lost 42lbs (19kg) and completed a challenge we set out to do, all in the space of 12 weeks.*

# BE CONSISTENT OR GO BACKWARDS

If you work from Monday to Friday, earn £100 a day and all your monthly bills add up to £1000, you will have an allowance of £1000 to spend or save.

If you reduce your working hours to only 2 ½ days a week you will only have enough money to pay your bills. If you reduce your work to one day a week, you will be £600 in debt of each month, and if you do not pay off your debt then you will start to receive **warnings.** Like letters coming through the door saying you owe money.

If you ignore these letters you will then receive bigger **warnings**, like debt collectors who will come and take away things that are worth the money you owe, or a letter telling you that you need to attend court. If you carry on ignoring these **warnings** you will lose your house, not have any money to buy food or clothes and be in a very bad situation, just because you didn't continue to work consistently.

Your body is the same. It is no good just doing a transformation course to lose some weight for 1 week, 4 weeks or 12 weeks, and then go back to your original lifestyle. You must consistently look after your body with consistent exercise and consistently good nutrition for as long as you live!

Funnily enough, if you start slacking, the same thing will happen as when you are in debt. Your body will give you **warnings.** Instead of having letters through the post, fat will start to appear. For men, it normally hits the lower belly and back, for women, it tends to go to the hips and thighs first.

If you start to ignore this, more **warnings** will appear. Your clothes will get tighter and you will have to start buying bigger clothes. You will get out of breath easier, your motivation will drop, and you may receive severe **warnings** of depression and anxiety.

Then, instead of debt collectors, it will be high blood pressure and the early signs of diabetes. Instead of being kicked out of your house and not being able to afford clothes and food, it will be diabetes, insulin resistance and the doctors telling you that you are going to have an early death.

If you want to escape an unhealthy, overweight body, don't expect a 12-week transformation course or an overnight operation to change your life. You must understand that you cannot just go back to the life you have been living. You are going to have to consistently exercise and eat healthily for a long time to escape an unhealthy, overweight body, and then continue for the rest of your life.

According to researchbriefings.parliament, in 2016, 61% of people were overweight in the UK alone and this number is increasing each year, which is insane. Now let's break it down.

What I think is more important to point out is the age at which people start to see an increase in obesity. Obesity levels start to rise in our late 20s and then there is another massive increase between the 30 and 40s, and obesity peaks the most between 45-65 years of age.

Let me remind you again, "Prevention is better than cure."

If you are younger than 40 and already have **warning signs**, start getting fit now and prevent yourself from becoming one of these statistics. If you are at the peak age for obesity and you are overweight then make it your mission to escape and join the happier side!

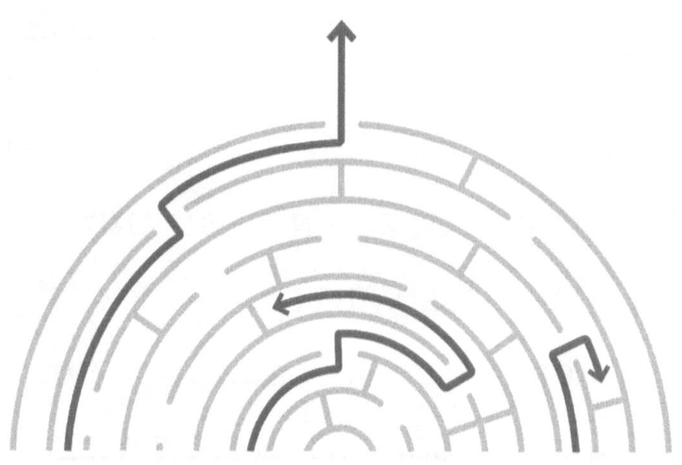

# CHAPTER 3

# OBSTACLE 3
# Knowledge

## WHAT IS KNOWLEDGE?

People say applied knowledge is power and it really is. As I have mentioned before, I thought I knew a great deal about fitness when I left the British Army. I thought I had all the answers, but I have learnt the value of constantly seeking to educate myself and improve my understanding so that I can better help people. There is always more to learn.

GIVE A POOR MAN A FISH AND

YOU FEED HIM FOR A DAY.

TEACH HIM TO FISH AND YOU GIVE

HIM AN OCCUPATION THAT WILL

FEED HIM FOR A LIFETIME.

# WHY IS KNOWLEDGE IMPORTANT?

One of the biggest mistakes and problems preventing people from losing weight is not knowing how to do it.

You may be sitting there thinking, I know what to do to lose weight, but I just don't have the motivation or there's no one around to give me a kick up the backside when I need it. Well, I'm afraid even this is due to you having a lack of knowledge, not knowing how to motivate yourself or not knowing how to give yourself a kick up the backside when you need it.

Give a poor man a fish and you feed him for a day. Teach him to fish and you give him an occupation that will feed him for a lifetime.

Weight loss is exactly the same. The only objective in losing weight is to get from A to B from being fat and unhealthy to looking and feeling fit and healthy.

I'm going to put this in a way that is easy to understand. Imagine that weight loss is a car journey from A to B. If you navigate with a map, it will only be a matter of time before you will no longer need a map or someone to guide you to complete that journey. On the flip side, if you are a passenger who spends the whole journey asleep and lets someone get you from A to B every time, you will always need someone to help you get to your destination.

# WHY YOU NEED TO LEARN TO DO IT YOURSELF

It's great to have a trainer, but you need to take the responsibility of learning and motivating yourself. If you are neither motivated nor determined, I would encourage you to join a personal training group. However, it is important to point out that a lot of people become emotionally attached to either a fitness group, class, gym or trainer.

What happens is, they sign up and make friends with the trainer or people in the class, gym or group. They also start feeling good because it's doing them good. Now that trainer, gym, class or group can only get them to a certain level. This is good, but for them to improve they need to get to the next stage. Emotions will control them, and they will become too scared to change so they will just stay at that level because they are comfortable.

The best way to understand this is to imagine the example of a boxer who starts as an amateur before becoming a professional. However, to progress as a professional boxer he will have to train with other professional boxers in order to improve. If he continues to train with amateur boxers, it will become extremely hard for him to get to the next stage, which is world-class. Just think, if you could be trained by Mike Tyson or go to your local gym, which route do you think would make you a better boxer?

You can't just jump to world-class, you have to work your way up, and escaping an unhealthy, overweight obese body is the same. It all depends on how much you want to change. If you want to lose weight, surround yourself with other people who are also trying to lose weight. Once you are one of the fittest people in that room go find another room where you're no longer the fittest.

It's how I became so fit. I spent 6 months training with what felt like ninjas (other recruits). By the end of 6 months, I was incredibly fit. But as I was getting fitter, so were the other ninjas and I was still trying to keep up with them.

I'm not expecting you to get to world-class level. But if you start in a beginner's class you must advance if you want to improve.

Now if this trainer decides to move, the gym shuts down or the fitness class/group stops, it prevents people from training or finding anything else to get them fitter because they were emotionally attached to that particular gym, trainer or group, and they never learned how to do it on their own.

This relates back to my point about learning to fish or being given the fish.

Personal trainers can be great because they will give guidance and teaching, whether that is in person or online. However, the quicker you can become self-motivated, self-disciplined and learn how to improve your body so that it is healthier (which is also a habit you can create) the better it will be. Once you have learnt to do all this, this is the point your life will change.

Then if you have a trainer it becomes a bonus. The first thing I tell my clients is I want to get them to the point where they'll never need to use me again (unless they want to). Now let me make that clear. I love training in a group, and I love having others train me, as it helps me to push that little bit harder. But I don't need anyone to push me. If I need to achieve a fitness level or body composition I can do that all myself and that is the discipline you should strive for.

**If you can focus on learning whilst you're changing and understand why you are doing certain exercises or why you eat certain food and what it does for your body, you will naturally become healthier.**

## KNOW WHAT THE DIET IS DOING TO YOUR BODY

The majority of clients that I take on tell me about all the diets they have tried and how they don't work, but most diets out there will work if they are taught correctly. The main reason they don't work for my clients, and probably for you, is because they haven't done it properly or have not stuck to it, and that is it.

Another big reason diets fail is because people do not understand the science and philosophy of the diet they are doing and will just eat what they have been told to eat without having a clue about what it does for their body. They are only focused on the result, not the process.

DO NOT LISTEN TO PEOPLE WHEN THEY SAY A CERTAIN DIET IS THE BEST FOR FAT LOSS. MOST DIETS ARE PRETTY GOOD, BUT THEY WORK IN DIFFERENT WAYS FOR DIFFERENT PEOPLE. YOU NEED TO FIND WHAT WORKS FOR YOU.

Let's take a keto diet, for example. A keto diet is a high fat, low carbohydrates diet, which allows your body to burn fat for fuel.

When doing a keto diet, the aim is to get into something called ketosis, which you do by consuming a certain amount of fat and reducing the carbohydrates you consume. When your carbohydrates are low enough, your body will start to burn the stored fat for fuel (putting you into ketosis).

Now even if you had just the smallest amount of carbohydrates, it could kick you out of ketosis. This is where a lot of people slip up. If you don't know what your diet is doing to your body, how can you expect to know when you are in or out of ketosis, let alone how to get back in?

Do you now start to understand the importance of knowledge?

Do not listen to people when they say a certain diet is the best for fat loss. Most diets are pretty good, but they work in different ways for different people. You need to find what works for you.

I highly recommend that you learn about the science and philosophy of it, and put yourself through a diet before deciding if it's right for you. Then pick a diet method (this could be keto, carb cycling, calorie counting, Palo, vegetarian, juice diet, intermittent fasting etc.) and spend 4-6 weeks trying it out 100%, whilst learning more about that diet and what it does for you. If you are on a journey to a healthier, fitter and happier lifestyle and the diet that you are testing is giving you results, I recommend sticking with that particular diet (even if you don't like it) until it stops giving you results. When you can put your hand on your heart and say that you are following the diet, but no longer getting results, you can then seek another diet to try and test.

It takes around 6 weeks to truly understand how well a certain diet will work for you or not, so stick with it.

On my The Weight is Over programme, I take my clients through multiple diet methods just so they can see what it does for their body and how well it works for their lifestyle.

How do I know this? Easy, if I gave one person a handful of nuts it would nourish their body. If I did the same to another person it would kill them. That little statement tells you that no one diet can fit all.

## MY STORY: LEARNING FOR MYSELF

My first step into the personal training world was a job at a gym called Pure Gym. While I was there, I was like a sponge, trying to learn anything and everything I could.

At that time, I was researching the keto diet (low-fat high carbs). I was given a negative opinion from a personal trainer colleague who I looked up to and respected, which put me off the diet. I even put off clients who would ask me about the keto diet.

KNOWLEDGE IS POWER.

START LEARNING.

But whilst I was researching about other nutrition methods, I kept seeing good research about the keto diet, and I wanted to find out more. I would never ask someone to do something I wouldn't do myself. Any diet I have ever recommended I have tried myself. I was so intrigued I thought I would give it a go.

I bought a plan off another personal trainer who was clued up about a keto diet and I was amazed about the outcome. From that moment on, I have taken advice with a pinch of salt unless I have personal experience of it. I would encourage you to do the same. If you are curious about something research it and then try it. See what it does for your body. Remember, we are all unique.

## BE OPEN TO BEING CORRECTED

Throughout this book, I refer to weight-loss because I have written it to help people who want to lose weight. But this is technically incorrect. It's not about losing weight; it's about losing fat and gaining as much muscle as possible. However, if I said this book was about "losing fat and gaining as much muscle as possible", most people would run for the hills, thinking I was trying to turn them into Arnold Schwarzenegger.

If you want to lose weight do not be scared of trying to build muscle, it's going to trim you down and make feel happy, confident and strong.

From now on, I will only be mentioning the technically correct term, which is 'fat loss'

Knowledge is power. Start learning.

# MY STORY: IGNORANCE

In Iraq, they would always put on little events throughout the year to keep us focused and entertained. I was asked to do a half marathon. I had 2 weeks' notice and didn't really change anything in my life. I didn't bother to learn how to train for a half marathon, although I had never done it before. When we did the event, I came 3rd out of 150 people.

The reason I am telling you that is because if I had known back then what I know now and actually combined the correct nutrition with the correct workouts. I could have easily won that race. However, I was too ignorant to want to learn because I thought I knew enough.

Just imagine being on a fat-loss journey. If you take the time to learn, you will be able to win first place in whatever it is you want to achieve.

# • KNOWLEDGE TASK •

It's very important that you start learning about how to become healthy because you can outsource a lot of things in your life. You can get someone to clean your car, build your house and wash your clothes. But you cannot outsource your health, you are the only one who is able to achieve that.

Now, in the last section, I talked a lot about nutrition to help you understand the importance of knowledge. However, knowledge is important in all aspects of health and fitness, so this task applies to both exercise and nutrition.

## Step 1

When you next start a nutrition or exercise plan, don't wait to learn about the exercise or nutrition method before starting. Start it first and then learn on the way. (However, do make sure you are physically capable of doing it. If you are unsure in the slightest, make sure your GP gives you the all-clear beforehand.)

## Step 2

Stick to the method religiously to get the most accurate outcome you can.

Step 3

Research the purpose of the method and what it's meant to do for your body, including the pros and cons. (Do not just type the name into Google and pick the first article or You-Tube video you can find. Find as many different resources as you can.)

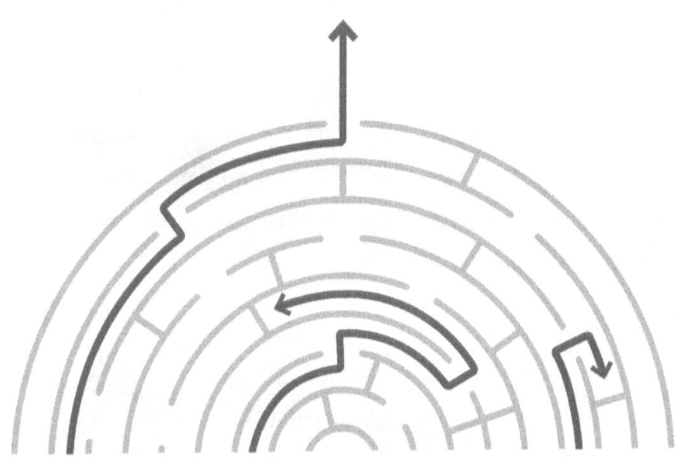

# OBSTACLE 4
## Motivation

## WHAT IS MOTIVATION?

Motivation is a reason or reasons for acting or behaving in a particular way. It is what keeps you going on your chosen course of action. You may be motivated by your trainer, your friends or family, as well as the inspirational stories of people you have never met. For example, watching a video that shows someone's transformational journey from being overweight to becoming healthy will motivate you to do whatever the person in the video did.

## WHY IS MOTIVATION IMPORTANT?

A fat-loss journey is not easy. You may be reading this and nodding your head. If you have ever tried going through a fat-loss journey, you know that you are going to hit so many hurdles along the way. These are not just exercise and nutrition, but also unsupportive peers (which could be your closest family and friends), special occasions, birthday parties, weddings, hen/stag dos, the list goes on…

You need to find a way to create motivation so that you will exercise when you need to, even when you don't want to, and you have the motivation and the willpower to say no if a friend offers you chocolate cake!

I learnt a very powerful tool from Tony Robbins. This is a routine he calls 'Priming' that he does every morning to get his mind and body in the best state it can be to perform the best he can each day. Priming helps you to stay motivated because what you do in the morning will have a big influence on the rest of your day.

Everyone can do this and it doesn't have to be the same for everyone. Personally, I do either one of two things. If I am working out on that day, I will get up early and the first thing I will do is workout before I do anything else. If I am not working out that day, I will brush my teeth as soon as I wake up, then drink 1 and a half pints of water, put my headphones in and listen to some music and go for a nice gentle walk for 2 miles.

After that, I'm motivated throughout the day. You can do the same too.

You also need little methods to do if you lose motivation throughout the day.

## PHASES IN PHASES

As you lose fat, you will be putting your body and mind under a lot of stress and you are going to have to fight different types of things, like frustration and temptations. At times, you will feel really low, and you might even feel depressed. You will be asking yourself why are you putting yourself through this misery? Is it worth it? Your mind will try and convince you to start again. It will be an endless battle and you'll end up fighting with yourself. The worse thing is, it never ends, and I like to call this 'phases in phases'. There are 4 phases.

**Phase 1** – Excited and motivated

**Phase 2** – Achieving results with the end in sight

**Phase 3** – Deflated and unmotivated

**Phase 4** – Revolution

Let's go through these phases. If, for example, you need to lose 70lb (32kg) and have just signed up to a fat-loss programme you really believe is going to change your life, here are the 4 phases you will face.

**You then enter Phase 1**, excited and motivated that you are actually doing something positive for yourself. You receive your instructions (this could be a nutrition plan and/or a weekly exercise guide) and stick to it religiously for the first couple of weeks. **Welcome to Phase 2.**

You start seeing results and have lost some fat. Your clothes are now looser and you really feel like it is the beginning of a new life, and then, all of a sudden, **Phase 3 appears!**

It is different for everyone. It may take 2 weeks or 6 weeks to enter phase 3, but you will hit it at some point. You may start missing all the things that you have cut out or reduced in your life, which could be the regular intake of sugar, or you see other people drinking alcohol and having fun and feel like you are missing out. Exercising starts to become a burden, your results start to slow down or stop altogether, and you don't feel like you are accomplishing anything. This is the stage when people quit, or they may continue exercising but the diet has gone right out of the window.

It is so important to regain focus and keep persisting. This stage can last between 2 days and 3 weeks and then, all of a sudden, phase 1 will reappear! (I have just come to this bit whilst writing this book. I'm currently on chapter 3, having written nearly 18,000 words, and I feel like I am in phase 3. I have so much left to write and I am questioning myself and I feel like quitting. But I have to continue. It happens to the best of us and if you are reading this, I was able to hit phase 4).

Yes, that's right, you go back to phase 1 and you will go through the cycle a few more times before you hit **Phase 4.** Now, this is not the end. It is different for different people. You may feel a revolution once you have lost 28lb (13kg) and can see a noticeable difference when you look in the mirror, or you can get to the top of the hill without being out of breath.

Did you notice how I said that you need to lose 70lb (32kg), but will feel a revolution at the 28lb (13kg) mark? This means you are motivated to go through all the phases again and again until you have hit your gold medal.

My first milestone in writing this book was completing the first draft. And my gold medal was finally publishing this book, which took 8 drafts.

The more you know about the hurdles, which could be nutrition, exercising, emotions, bad habits, the easier it is going to be to overcome them. If you do not understand them, I can guarantee when you hit enough hurdles, your fat-loss journey will stop, and you will end up back in the body that has made you feel trapped.

BEING HEALTHY IS NOT ABOUT

NUMBERS, IT'S A FEELING THAT

YOU ARE FIT AND HEALTHY.

# WHY SCALES AND STATS WILL NOT MOTIVATE YOU

Stay away from the scales. Unless you understand why you are using them, they will be a burden throughout your journey and demotivate you even when you are succeeding. I have seen many people get upset after weighing themselves in front of others during my group training programmes, because they haven't lost as much as someone else. It's crazy because they have also lost weight.

In 2017, we were 6 weeks into another group training programme I ran, and it was weighing and taping day. One client called Jill had lost 21lbs (9kg) and 4 inches off her waist. Another called Rachel had lost 10lbs (4.5kg) and 4 inches off her waist. Now, as you can see, they both lost the same amount of inches off their waist. However, Rachel was devastated that she hadn't lost as much weight as Jill had, even though she had done just as well. She felt like she had failed because the scales didn't say what she wanted them to say.

From that day on, I stopped using scales and created the health level table (on page 9) for any future clients, and it is the only thing I will relate to, NOT the scales.

There are a few things I want to go through when it comes to scales:

1. Understanding when you should stop worrying about the scales

2. Weight-loss patterns

3. Becoming addicted to numbers

4. What to focus on instead

## 1. Understanding when you should stop worrying about the scales

I have mentioned this briefly before but if you are seeking weight loss then gaining muscle and losing fat is more important than trying to get the numbers on the scales to drop.

Muscle is denser than fat, so if you have 10lbs (4.5kg) of fat in one hand and 10lbs of muscle in another, the muscle is roughly 18% more dense than the fat. You could have 13lbs (6kg) of muscle and it will still look smaller than 10lbs (4.5kgs) of fat. Now if you were to put 10lbs of fat in a concealed container and 13lbs of muscle in another concealed container, the 13lbs of muscle would look smaller but it will be heavier. This is where people go wrong because all they worry about is the numbers.

Now, I understand if you are 5ft and 280lb (127kg) of mostly fat, then it is clear that you need to lose weight and get the numbers on the scale down. However, there will come a point the scales are no longer necessary, which leads me on to the **weight-loss pattern.**

# 2. Weight-loss patterns

Let's hypothetically say I have someone who is 5ft, 280lbs (127kg) and a size 22. Within the first month, they can easily lose a minimum of 14lbs (6kg) and 2 dress sizes. Then, 2 weeks later they may put on a few pounds but the inches on their body will shrink. After a few months, they will lose a 14 more pounds and another dress size, so now they are 252lbs (114kg) and size 16/18. A couple of weeks go by and they put on a few pounds (of muscle) and the scales will increase, but once again, the inches on their body will shrink.

These patterns will continue until they are at a healthy size of say 10/12. They may be 140lbs (63.5kg) at this point, and if they want to take it a step further and get down to a size 8/10, they should concentrate on creating more muscle whilst stripping fat. What happens is their weight will no longer drop but go back up to maybe 154lbs (70kg) but they will drop to size 8.

To summarise, if someone is doing it properly, the number on the scales will go down and up throughout their journey, but the inches on their body will continually shrink.

A lot of people will focus on the scales and start doing the wrong things as soon as they see the numbers increase, like stop eating and other crazy stuff so their body no longer gets enough nutrition to be able to improve.

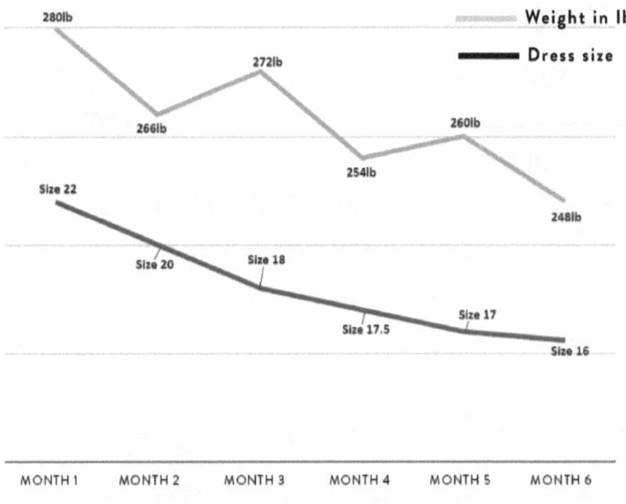


WOMEN'S DRESS SIZE VS WOMEN'S WEIGHT

## 3. Becoming addicted to numbers

This is where it can get dangerous, because the fitter you get, the more obsessed you become with the numbers (on the scales, the inches on your body etc.). If the numbers aren't improving, or at least aren't improving as much as someone that you compare yourself with, you will get disheartened very quickly.

Being healthy is not about numbers, it's a feeling that you are fit and healthy.

## 4. What to focus on instead

Okay, so everyone loves to see results and just how much they have improved, so a great little way to do this without any numbers is by measuring yourself with string. Get a piece and wrap it around your belly. Then cut it off where it meets and label that bit of string 'belly with the date'. Repeat this for your bum, both of your legs and arms, and then repeat this process every month. You will then be able to pair the strings together to see the difference.

## • MOTIVATION TASK •

A simple motivation task.

I want you to try my motivational tool that I use daily. This task aims to motivate you and get you inspired before you even start your day.

### Step 1

Think of a goal; for example, it might be to lose a certain amount of fat.

### Step 2

Tomorrow, I want you to wake up an hour earlier than you would normally to start your day. If you cannot do it tomorrow make sure you do this within the next 7 days.

### Step 3

The first thing you should do when you wake up is brush your teeth, drink a big glass of water and go for a nice gentle walk (for at least 30 minutes). I also want you to listen to something that is inspiring for your particular goal. For example, if you are trying to lose fat, you could listen (not watch) to one of my educational videos on YouTube (YouTube channel: Chris Marco Flores) that talks about how to escape a body that you feel trapped in, or you could listen to a really inspiring story about someone who has lost a lot of fat, in which they talk about how they did this and how it has changed their life. You can find this kind of story all over the internet.

## Step 4

Write down how motivated you feel once you have finished your walk.

The first time you do it, you might not feel great, as you are disrupting what you normally do, so…

## Step 5

Do this for 7 consecutive days before making a judgement, and see how much more productive you are throughout the day.

Now this works really well for me and it is something I have been doing for a very long time, but remember, you must find a way that will motivate you. Once you have found how to do it, make sure you turn it into a habit.

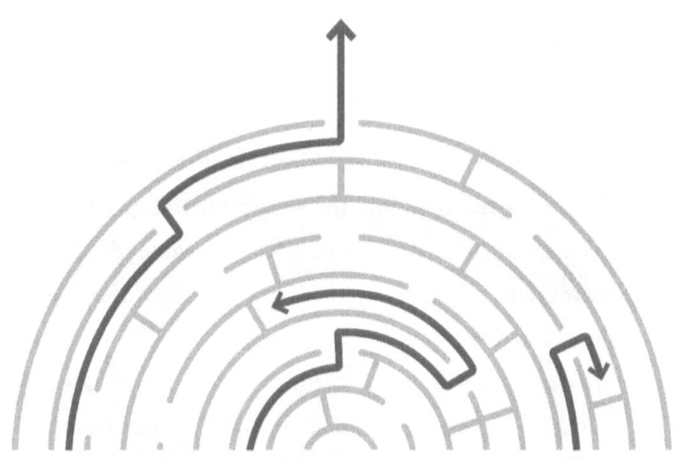

# OBSTACLE 5
## Lack of support

### WHAT IS SUPPORT?

Support is a tool that helps you to achieve your goal of trying to escape an unhealthy, overweight body. There are all sorts of support tools that will aid you. It is always easier to achieve something if the people around you can support you.

This can come in different forms, but I'd like to focus on 2 key tools.

1.  **Fat-loss Programmes:** These are either online or offline, and will outline exactly what you need to do and when you need to do it. If you follow the programme's tools step by step, the support of the programme will help you to achieve what you desire.

2.  **Environment:** People underestimate the power of their environment and the support it will give them. If you spent every day surrounded by people who had no intention of exercising at all and only ate unhealthy, processed food all day long, what would you be likely to do? However, if you spent every day surrounded by people who exercise daily and eat incredibly healthily and live and breathe health and fitness, talking about what healthy and delicious meals they make, what would you be likely to do? Which environment do you think would support you the most when you are trying to escape an unhealthy, overweight body?

## WHY IS SUPPORT IMPORTANT?

Your peers will make you either fail or succeed. You may have heard this many times before, but who you surround yourself with will influence your success or failure. If you hang around with people who don't eat anything healthy, fail to exercise and have no desire to be healthy, while you are trying to go on a

IF YOU ARE STRUGGLING AND
FINDING IT HARD TO ACHIEVE
WHAT YOU DESIRE, IT IS ALWAYS
GOOD TO HAVE A MENTOR WHO HAS
HAD SUCCESS WITH WHATEVER YOU
ARE TRYING TO ACHIEVE. I LOOK AT
MENTORS LIKE THE CHEAT CODES
FOR LIFE.

journey to lose fat, they will not support or influence your success. They will only influence your failure.

I've had clients whose partners encouraged them to do the things I have asked them and joined in, even if they didn't need to lose any fat themselves. These clients always succeeded.

I have also had clients whose partners and family did the opposite and would not join in the exercise and refused to eat healthy meals. The majority of these clients did not succeed, and this really saddens me.

Another great saying that I love is:

***If you don't believe in yourself, find people who do and surround yourself with them and get rid of anyone who doesn't.***

I like to think that I made that one up.

If you are struggling and finding it hard to achieve what you desire, it is always good to have a mentor who has had success with whatever you are trying to achieve. I look at mentors like the cheat codes for life.

However, although there are mentors who really care about you deep down and want you to succeed, there are others who just want your money. Make sure you pick wisely.

# MY STORY: MY HOUSEMATES

Let me tell you a little story about when I was living in a house share in Cardiff, and everyone in the house had a visible six-pack. It was one of my most memorable summers, but it came with a price.

I moved into this house in 2014 unsure of what to expect. Everyone was new to house-sharing and not one of us knew each other beforehand. At the beginning of the summer, there were 3 people, Elliot (a science teacher) Abby (a retail assistant) and me (a personal trainer).

Abby and I were very much into our fitness. I had a lot of scientific knowledge about becoming fit. Abby had done a lot of fitness, but didn't know too much science behind it, and Elliot knew he should get serious about fitness, but didn't really have any intention to start and just wanted to enjoy life.

I created and put myself through a lot of fitness plans throughout 2014 and I would come home each night after work between 8pm and 10pm and cook all the food that I needed to consume, ready for the next day.

Abby and Elliot would both ask what I was doing regarding my nutrition. As I explained, I inspired them and naturally, they ended up creating their own nutrition plans. As Abby and I trained so much Elliot ended up joining us, despite his initial reluctance.

> THE MORE YOU CAN LEARN TO CHANGE YOUR LIFESTYLE, THE GREATER YOUR CHANCE OF SUCCESS.

I remember at the beginning of the summer, Elliot told me that genetics has a lot to play with why he couldn't get abs and he thought he never would. But by the end of the summer, all 3 of us had great visible abs and it was all down to the influence of being around the right people.

So, if you are reading this Elliot, I told you so, ha! P.S. I hope you are well.

So that was the good influence we got from hanging around each other and inspiring each other and working out together. But there was also a bad side to it.

We created a friendship through drinking at the weekends. There would be weekends when one of us really didn't want to go out, but we would because everyone else was, and we couldn't help but go and get drunk together. At the time, this seemed like the greatest fun ever but it took its toll, of course. We did it so much that it affected us financially and some of us mentally, as we were becoming both broke and depressed.

As we'd created such a great friendship on a lifestyle of working and partying, we had to break the pattern if we were to improve. The best way for us to do this was to move out and remove ourselves from the environment that we had created, regardless of how much we liked each other. By doing so our mental health and financial situations improved instantly.

This is what you need to do with your environment if you want a better chance of succeeding.

# THE DANGERS OF UNSUPPORTIVE PEOPLE

It will be the same for you. If you hang around people who enjoy drinking, love fast food and hate the thought of exercising, you will have very little support when you try to improve yourself. Worse still, when you start improving or looking better, people may become silently jealous and question why you are doing what you are doing and encourage you to stop.

Even if they are not jealous, they may miss you going out with them, whether you're skipping your weekly Pizza Hut date or drinks after work, and encourage you to break your healthy habit to join them out "just one time". This is not them being mean, but it's how they have built a friendship with you and they want their companion back.

As sad as it may sound, it is hard to find supportive people who actually want to help you to escape an unhealthy, overweight body, and easier to find people who try and knock you off the horse.

I understand that it is a big deal asking you to stop hanging around with people who have been your friends for a lifetime. It sounds harsh, but if they are not supporting you or are not going in the same direction as you, it is very important that you do.

The more you can learn to change your lifestyle, the greater your chance of success.

It doesn't have to be forever, but if you are unhappy and obese then you need to ensure that for a period of time you are only spending time with people who are going in the same direction as you and can support you on your journey.

You will need to ditch friends who drink in the evening and after work and find people who exercise after work, or ditch people who focus on the next festival and find people who focus on the next fitness event. You get my drift.

Let's put it into percentages:

- 60% of the people you hang around with should be people who you want to be like – people fitter and healthier than you.

- 30% of people you hang around with should be going in the same direction as you, and be trying to escape their overweight, unhealthy body. (So that you are not doing it alone.)

- 10% of people you hang around with should be in a worse position than you are so that you can help bring them along and teach them what you learn.

## A NOTE ON THE DISBELIEVERS

Be careful about spending time with overweight people who are not motivated to change. They have given up and don't want you to change because that would force them to do something about their situation. They may be in denial and tell you that 'being big is beautiful' or that being beautiful is about the person inside of you regardless of what you look like.

The fact is, being overweight is not healthy, and the 'being big is beautiful' role models are only encouraging people not to get healthy. I can guarantee that a lot of plus-size models want to change deep down.

It's 100% possible to break away from a weight and body you're not happy with and live a life you dream of. However, if you are in a position that does not make you happy, it is not going to happen overnight. If you are an overweight person the bigger you become the harder and longer it will take to reverse, but not impossible.

Don't do it for others, do it for you, but be open and you will be surprised about how many people will want to help and support you.

If you are around people who are negative towards you when you are trying to achieve your goals then my advice would be to get rid of them completely!

## FRIENDS + FAMILY = PROBLEMS

There will be problems you face along the way with your family and friends. Even if you do change your identity to some degree and also change the people you hang around with, there are going to be those who you cannot avoid. This could be your colleagues at work or your family at home. So here are some tips on dealing with unavoidable negative people from my own experiences and those of my clients. I hate to be negative but sometimes you have to be, and if you consciously know this, it's going to be easier to tackle.

Let's break it down:

1. Family

2. Others (colleagues/clients)

3. Silent haters

## 1. Family

*Kids*

If you have kids, a little part of your relationship with them may have been built around certain foods. For example, you might end the night with a hot chocolate together or have a film night once a week which involves lots of naughty eating (it could be different for you and your family). If you are trying to escape an overweight, unhealthy body, this will eventually have to change (you can come back to your naughty nights and drinks when you are at your goal, but for a period, you will have to stop or substitute them for a healthier option).

Your kids will not understand why you have suddenly stopped, and it might be hard for you as a parent to stop as it's how you've bonded together. It will also be hard to try and explain what you are doing and why you can't have certain things. At first, your kids might not understand, but if you teach them about what you are doing and they see you are changing physically and emotionally by cutting out the bad stuff, you will be surprised how much you will inspire your kids to make healthier choices. They will be proud of you.

I know this from first-hand experience. My previous partner's daughter, who I still consider to be my step-daughter, always eats junk with me. She knows how much I love chocolate, and when I put myself on a plan and cut it all out, she was very confused and would try and tempt me every day. I remember one day she put this chocolate cake in front of me and tried to over-exaggerate by saying, "It's double chocolate, topped with triple chocolate and inside it has all types of chocolate that melts in your mouth, go on just have one bite." When I turned it down, the surprise on her face was priceless. I have heard her tell her friends about it. She never said anything, but you could tell she was inspired.

*Partners*

This may sound shocking, but often when I train people they start getting amazing results, and tell me how their partners are trying to sabotage their efforts. The partners do this by telling them they look great now and can stop losing weight, or by telling them they prefer them looking bigger. In the most extreme cases, they may threaten to leave them if they carry on going to the gym or improving themselves.

"

NO MATTER HOW MUCH YOU HAVE PAID FOR WHATEVER COURSE YOU ARE DOING TO IMPROVE YOURSELF, I ENCOURAGE YOU TO TEACH IT TO AS MANY PEOPLE AS POSSIBLE, BECAUSE WHEN YOU TEACH YOU ALSO LEARN.

"

This is pure jealousy and stems from a fear that you may run off with someone else.

I always say you can never give advice on someone else's relationship, but if someone is telling you they want you to stop improving your health and fitness because they don't like it, you must stick up for yourself, regardless of how close you are or how long you have known them.

If you don't you are letting someone else determine your happiness. If they love you enough then they should support what makes you happy.

A very good way to do this is to educate them because they may not understand what you are doing and how you are doing it. Educating them is a great way to get your partner on your side, although it doesn't always work, unfortunately.

Sadly, I have had clients who couldn't stick up for themselves and guess what happened? When I bumped into them a few months down the road, they had gone back to square one to please their partners. Do not let your partner be a hurdle.

## 2.Others (colleagues/clients)

Everyone is different and every work environment will be different, but the concept will be the same. You will have CCs who will support you and be intrigued by what you are doing and keen to learn more.

No matter how much you have paid for whatever course you are doing to improve yourself, I encourage you to teach it to as many people as possible, because when you teach you also learn.

When you have CCs who are intrigued, talk about it as much as you can. Help them as much as you can, and they will then become your new best friends.

You will also have to face CCs who are jealous and try everything they can to put you off by doing little things like bringing in biscuits or chocolate treats for everyone to have or try and encourage you to do stuff you shouldn't. They may also make fun of you and try and put you down. You will need to grow thicker skin towards these people or just punch them in the face! (Not advisable in the office!) I'm only joking, don't punch them in the face, but stick up for yourself.

If they offer you anything you know you shouldn't have, put it in the bin in front of them. If it is wine, pour it down the drain as this will show them you are serious. If you do it long enough they will stop.

## 3. Silent haters

These are the worst because they are normally the closest people to you and when you tell them what you are doing they will sound so supportive and encouraging, but they will drop little hints to put you off. If you don't believe me now, you will know what I am talking about when you come across it.

For example, you tell them you are on a fat-loss course and they say something like, "How long are you going to give it before you give it up?" Stick up for yourself, explain how serious you are about it and if they can't get on board, get rid of their negativity and start surrounding yourself with others you want to be like.



Figure out the people who support you the most.

### Step 1

Write down a list of all the people you interact with and write down a number between 1-10.

1= indicates that this person is very unsupportive.

10= indicates that this person is very supportive. (These are the people you want to hang around with more whilst on your journey.)

### Step 2

Figure out who are the 5 people you interact with the most. This doesn't just have to be in person, you may interact over the phone or online.

## Step 3

Take the time to make sure the 5 people who you interact with the most are a 7 or more on the supportive scale.

Remember, if someone is a 1, it doesn't mean they don't want the best for you. You could have built a great relationship with them by doing things that stop you from achieving a certain goal and they want the relationship to remain like that.

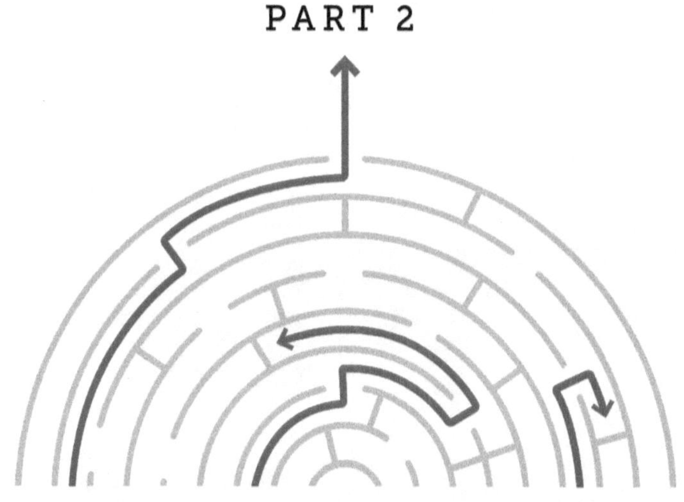

# THE 5 VITAL ACTIVITIES

# INTRODUCTION TO PART 2

If you are looking for long-term fat loss results, this is the most important part of the book for you. In this part of the book, I would like to share with you the 5 Vital Activities. These, I believe, are the foundation of any health and fitness challenge no matter how advanced you are, whether your challenge is a 5km run or an Ironman. The 5 Vital Activities are Mindset, Challenges, Exercise, Nutrition, Planning and Preparation.

Without implementing any of the 5 Vital Activities, you are winging it. Your results will be unpredictable or poor.

Without the right **Mindset**, you have no clarity over what you are trying to achieve or why, so this is where we'll start.

Without a **Challenge** in place, you cannot see where you are going. Putting a challenge in place gives you something to aim for, just like when you put an exact location into a sat nav and you know what tracks to stay on.

**Exercise** and **Nutrition** are two separate activities, so it's important to go in-depth on both, but the principles are the same. If you don't know why you are doing what you are doing, you can compromise your results. For example, you don't ever see a body builder who is training to get bigger train with a marathon runner, because if he/she did, there is not a chance in hell they would get any bigger. In fact, he/she would get smaller.

If the marathon runner tried to eat like a body builder, he/she would also compromise his/her results. Nutrition is fuel and you need to fuel yourself in different ways for different goals.

Lastly, **Planning and Preparation**. If you take the time to plan and prepare, it takes away all the guessing, completely! If you are trying to lose fat, you must plan and calculate exactly what you need to do to lose a certain amount of fat each week. If you are planning to strengthen certain muscles in your body, you need to plan exercises that will do that.

To give you an example of how useful the 5 Vital Activities are, I'll tell you about Andrew, a client and now a good friend. When I met Andrew, he was 41 years old and a UK size XL (42 inches) shirt size. All he wanted to do was to lose weight, but I dug a little deeper and implemented the Vital Activities.

## MINDSET

He wanted to lose weight so he could be confident enough to go to his Christmas party and feel proud, happy and comfortable while he was there.

## CHALLENGE

To fit into a UK size medium (38 inches) white shirt for his work Christmas party, which he didn't normally have the confidence to attend. That day I told him to go and buy a UK size medium (38 inches) white shirt and hang it where he could see it every morning to remind him of the goal he was trying to achieve.

## EXERCISE

**Month 1** – Cardio to help him understand that he could do more than he could imagine. The fitter he was at cardio, the better he would be at lifting weights.

**Month 2** – Hypertrophy weight lifting to increase the muscle in his body.

**Month 3** – Cardio + endurance weight training to help strip as much fat as possible whilst retaining as much muscle as we could.

## NUTRITION

**Month 1** – I put him on a plan that I like to call Keep It Simple, which helps people go from poor nutrition to good nutrition with very little stress.

**Month 2** – A well-known method called Carb Cycling which helps to retain muscle tension whilst stripping fat and boosting the function of the metabolism.

**Month 3** – On the third month, I wanted to strip as much fat as possible. From experience, I know that one of the best ways to do this is to completely switch up the diet. I find this shocks the body and gives rapid results. I also put him on a keto diet for 4 weeks.

## PLANNING AND PREPARATION

I put plans together so he knew exactly when he was training, exactly what training he would be doing and what he would be eating for the whole three months. He had the whole 3 months planned out, so there was no guessing at all.

The results: I remember Andrew ringing me just before his Christmas party. I asked him whether the shirt he had bought all those months ago now fitted.

Andrew replied, "I tried the shirt on the other day Chris and it didn't fit. I had to go buy another shirt and they'd sold out of white so I had to buy a blue." My heart sank, I didn't say anything because he had worked so hard. He continued, "By the way Chris, I had to go and buy a UK size small (36 inches)."

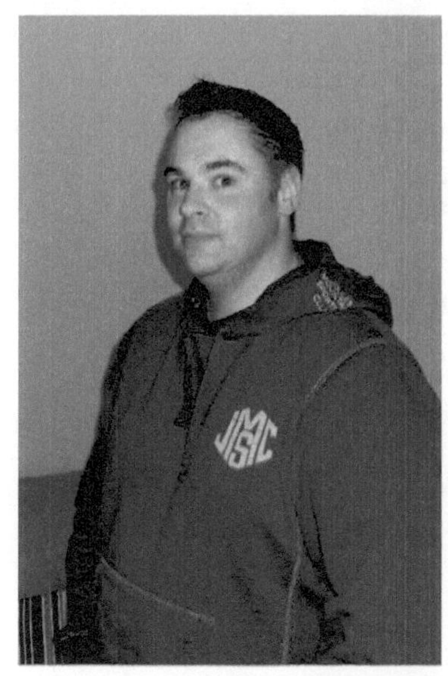

BEFORE

AFTER

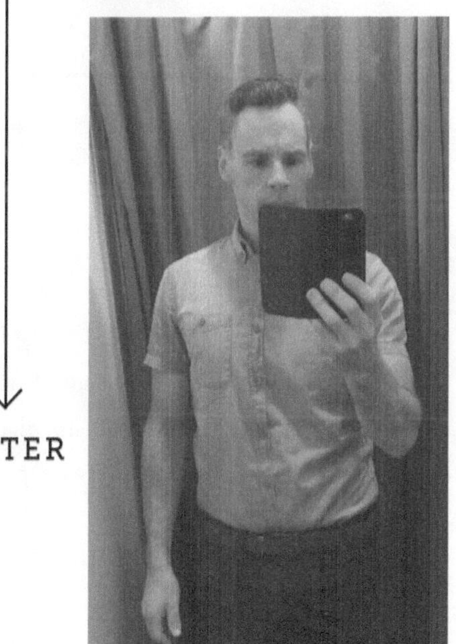

I couldn't believe it, we were both over the moon. He had absolutely smashed his goal of getting to a medium size and was now a small. This is because we had the structure of the 5 Vital Activities.

## The formula of success

Scientists create formulas and formulas create outcomes. When you change, and add or take away from that formula, it creates a different outcome. The 5 Vital Activities can be thought of as a formula – you will need each part of the equation.

If formulas change, they have different outcomes:

Car + fuel = a moving car

Hot water + coffee = hot coffee

Change the formula and you change the outcome:

Car + no fuel = no moving car

Hot water + tea bag = hot tea

Escaping an unhealthy, overweight body is the same. There are formulas and each one will create different outcomes. To escape, you have to put a formula in place that is going to change your lifestyle. Too many people replace a few things but not others.

Imagine that this is your formula:

**Bad nutrition (takeaways, fizzy drinks) + alcohol + no exercise = weight gain.**

People fail by either adding to their original formula or only changing one or two things.

**Bad nutrition + alcohol + no exercise + fat burning tablets**

Or

**Replacement shakes + alcohol + no exercise**

Either one of these formulas may help people to lose a little bit of weight very quickly or a lot of weight very quickly, and because they have lost weight they then go back to their original lifestyle, so it's only a matter of time before they end back where they started. However, they will end up putting on weight again because they haven't positively changed their lifestyle. Or the methods where you don't need to change your lifestyle, like having an operation in hospital to pump some fat out. Although you think your weight-loss battle is all over, you haven't learned how to improve your day-to-day health, so you don't actually change your lifestyle. You just add to your current lifestyle formula and when you come out of the operation, you just continue as normal and end up back at square one.

Some people do not change the formula enough and don't lose anything at all and will always blame everything else.

The simplest formula you need to use for the rest of your life is:

Good nutrition + exercise + time = escaping fat-loss forever

However, there are ways to strengthen this formula and increase your chances of success. I've now got more than 10 years' experience of helping people to escape an unhealthy, overweight body for good, and I've found this is by far the best formula I have created. It will give you nothing but success, so don't add or take away anything from it.

## Mindset + Challenges + Exercise + Nutrition + Planning and Preparation

As you can tell from this book, each of these factors can also be broken down. If you take something away from the formula, it becomes weaker and if you ever add to it then you might compromise the whole system.

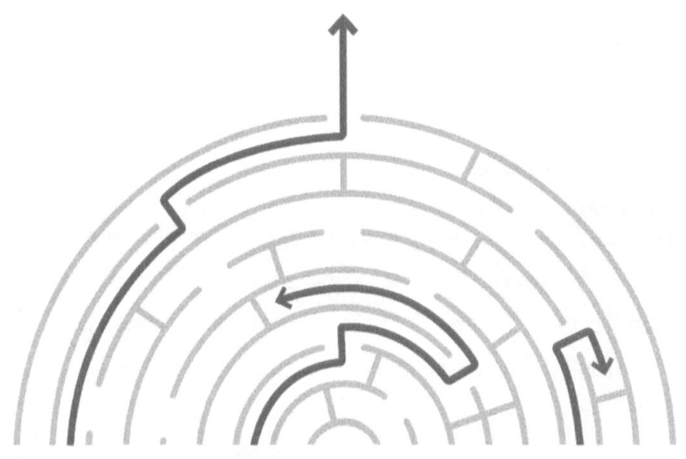

# VITAL ACTIVITY 1
## Mindset

## WHAT IS MINDSET?

Mindset is your mental attitude. It is the way you think about and approach a challenge. This is something we worked on a lot in the Army because your mindset has the power and ability to make sure that you stay focused enough to achieve what you desire, regardless of what gets in the way. To get results you need to focus. Your mindset is the best place to start.

People talk about getting in the right mindset but then they don't actively take action to get in the right mindset. There is a big difference.

## WHY IS MINDSET A VITAL ACTIVITY?

Any challenge is not easy, so we need a strong, powerful and positive mindset if we're going to stick at it, rather than quit as soon as the going gets tough. Far too many people quit when they don't see instant results.

For example, most people want a level of wealth and lots of money. This is not because they can look at bits of paper with faces on them (notes), it's because of the feeling and freedom they think it is going to give them. You wanting to lose weight is the same.

Let's hypothetically say you are 280lbs (127kg) and your dream is to be 154lbs (70kg). It's not really about the number on the scales, it is the feeling and freedom you think it's going to give you. Maybe it's the freedom to wear a bikini without worrying about what others think, knowing you can run 5 miles or not being the fattest person in the photos.

To break the back of this challenge, you need a strong mindset because you have to push yourself hard enough for long enough and overcome all your barriers. When you have reached the top of the mountain, you haven't hit your dream goal, but you have come far enough to know that deep down nothing is going to stop you and you are on the way to becoming the person you want to be!

If you are overweight and trying to escape, this will be the hardest challenge and journey of your life! It may take 1 year or possibly 2, depending on how overweight you are and how far you need to go. Now, 2 years sounds like a long time to suffer, but it's a lot better than a lifetime of being trapped in a body that makes you suffer every day of your life.

You are going to have to put yourself through physical and mental pain that will make you want to quit nearly every day. Just remember that you are not the only one who has been in this position; others like you have managed to break free and the only person who is going to stop you is you!

## WHAT HAPPENS IF YOU DON'T GET YOUR MINDSET RIGHT?

This element is very easily missed. Even if people understand they need to be in the right mindset, they will very rarely do this consciously. Getting into the right mindset is not taught enough. As a result, people think that by just saying they will lose weight and thinking about it will be enough.

It's like saying on a Sunday night, "I'm going on holiday tomorrow," and then just spontaneously turning up at the airport with no idea about where you are going or how long for. The majority of people who go on holiday plan it months in advance. They will spend hours, days or even weeks deciding what kind of holiday they want and researching the best places to go. After that, they find out how much it costs and then figure out how they will afford it. After that, they are then fully prepared and in the right mindset. They know what they are doing, when they will do it, how long they are doing it and why.

That is why a lot of people fail to lose weight. One day they will say to themselves, "Right, I'm going to lose weight starting Monday," and that is it. They don't do any real planning or preparation, let alone getting their mindset right. And when it comes to the Monday, a lot of people don't even start, or if they do, they can't stick with their mission for very long.

## MY STORY: MINDSET

Mindset is a muscle, so the more you train it the stronger it becomes. I could tell you many stories when I was in dangerous situations and I had to have a clear, focussed and determined mind, but I think 2 little stories will help you the most. They are both about the training I had to undergo before entering the British Army and the US Army.

To qualify to be a soldier in the British or US Army, you have to complete a phase of training (6 months for the British, which is called basic training, and 3 months for the US, which is called Boot Camp), where they train you up. In both cases, they test you on different skills that you have acquired throughout the training. For example, they test you on your physical abilities, your shooting skills and all sorts of combat-ready skills tests.

If you don't pass, you are not allowed to continue to the next stage of training, and if you fail too many times, you are asked to leave and will not be allowed to continue to be qualified as a soldier.

As I explain this next part, I want you to relate this to a journey that you are trying to accomplish yourself. For example, you might be trying to lose 8 dress sizes, whereas in this example, I was trying to complete Army training to become a soldier.

The first Army I tried to join was the British Army. It was the beginning of my journey, I was 16 years old and I was about to face 6 months of basic training. Before I started basic training, I had no clue about what to expect. I knew they were going to make us do a lot of exercise, but I had no clue what a normal day would look like.

Everyone I spoke to told me that it's one of the hardest things you will ever do, and that I should prepare. I was under a lot of pressure and worried sick that I wasn't going to have a strong enough mindset to be able to complete it. I was worried that I might have to quit before the end as I was the youngest. When the day came, and I had to get on a 12-hour train journey to Catterick (which was the basic training barracks for the British Infantry), you can just imagine how weak my mind felt. I thought I was going to endure six months of torture.

I wasn't wrong. The whole six months felt like torture. It was by far the hardest thing I had ever encountered. I remember dreaming that I was back at home enjoying time with my friends and then I would wake up in Catterick about to start another day of pain. That was the worst start to the day.

It was so hard; my mind was telling me to quit every day. On three occasions, I came very close to quitting and I even packed my bag to run away twice. The only reason I was able to stay focused was due to everyone else I was with, and my dad. I created very good friendships with the boys I trained with and every time I wanted to quit, the boys would get together to talk me into staying as they were going through the same thing as I was. Then, when the boys couldn't talk me through, I would ring my dad and he would tell me, 'Give it two more days, and if you feel the same then leave,' even though he would say the same thing two days later.

I was only able to complete the training and become a British soldier because of my environment and the people supporting me. If I had been on my own, I would have probably left.

Six years after the British Army basic training, I joined the American Army Boot Camp, which lasted 3 months. This time I was very well prepared, both mentally and physically, as I already had my previous Army experience under my belt and I now knew what I was about to endure. On the first day, my mindset was good, sharp and strong. It didn't matter what they were going to chuck at me, there was no way, in my mind, that I was not going to pass. Throughout the whole 3 months, I didn't need anyone's shoulder to cry on, I was far too mentally

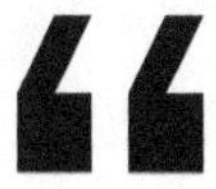

I'M A BIG FAN OF SAYINGS AND THIS IS ANOTHER FAVOURITE OF MINE: 'GET COMFORTABLE BEING UNCOMFORTABLE.'

focused and determined. This strong mindset paid off and I passed with flying colours.

It's the same with any journey that you endure, especially when it comes to trying to lose fat. When you first start, it's hard and until you get over the first big hurdles, you are going to want to quit every day until you have achieved a level of success that allows you to get into a mindset where you become unstoppable.

## MINDSET AND EXERCISE

Breaking free from an unhealthy, overweight body boils down to two elements – exercise and nutrition. If you eat the right food and the right amount of it for a long enough period and combine it with the right exercise, you can say goodbye to an unhealthy, overweight body. However, you need to realise that in both elements, your mind is what will give up before anything else.

Your mind is also a muscle, so the more you train it, the stronger it will become. You need to push your mind to a point where you feel uncomfortable.

If you push your body and mind past the comfort zone and into an uncomfortable position, you become stronger. This is the position you need to get to regularly if you are to change.

Some people will go to the gym three times a week but then do the same thing each time they go, or if they do change, their intensity will always stay the same. This person will then be confused as to why they are not changing.

Our body adapts and gets used to things you repeat. If you go to a gym and do three different types of classes a week but the intensity remains the same, your body will adapt.

If you are not used to pushing yourself past a point where your body feels uncomfortable, your mind will encourage you to stop and go back to where it feels comfortable.

For example, say you do 10 push-ups every day and then one day you try to do 30. As soon as you get past 10, your mind will start trying to convince you that you cannot do any more or that you have done enough for today and you can try to do 30 another day.

I'm a big fan of sayings and this is another favourite of mine: 'Get comfortable being uncomfortable.'

When it comes to exercise, you should try and get to the uncomfortable feeling and push yourself a minimum of 3 times a week. Feeling uncomfortable is not a sign to stop. This is the point that is going to make you change.

## MINDSET AND NUTRITION

Nutrition is even harder. If you crave sugar or/and caffeine when you start cutting it out, you will have mental battles with those temptations throughout your daily life. You'll see adverts for McDonald's, KFC, and coffee shops offering free shots.

Even when you are watching TV at home, you'll see adverts for new chocolate bars or refreshing sugary drinks. Even the pizza shop will text your phone to tempt you with their offers.

It becomes extremely hard to resist, but the more you learn to the easier it becomes. If you always give in, then you will always give in.

## MINDSET AND GYMS

This also relates to going to places where you feel uncomfortable. For example, you may not be very comfortable going to a gym. You may think that you want to lose fat before joining because you are self-conscious. This completely defeats the purpose. For you to become fitter, you need to exercise and going to a gym will help you do that. Far too many people are worried about perceived challenges, such as thinking, 'If I go to the gym everyone will look at me and I'll feel really unfit.' When people go to the gym so they can become fit. They don't wait until they are fit to join. People don't go to the gym so they can watch other people, they are too busy doing their own workout. Or another perceived challenge is, 'I won't know what to do in a gym.' Again, this is no problem as 90% of gyms will offer you demonstrations or inductions before starting.

Be brave and change your mindset from "I'm too overweight to go to a gym. I wouldn't know what to do anyhow" to "I'm going to join a gym to lose fat. I will book an induction and ask them how to use the equipment."

A gym is not the only way you can become fit or lose fat. There are a few places I would say you need to be fit to join, rather than join to become fit. Remember, once you are the fittest person in the room go to the next one. So you will need to be fit enough to join some rooms, otherwise, it could put you off fitness very quickly.

If one of the following is not offering a beginner's class and you haven't done fitness for a long time, I would seek other options to build your fitness levels up first.

- CrossFit

- Boxing (not boxercise)

- MMA (mix martial arts or any type of martial arts)

- Any high-level sports

- Triathlon training

Now, I know I said you need to push and make yourself feel uncomfortable, but if you are just starting out, find a fitness class first or a course suitable for beginners.

## HAVE A CARING MINDSET TOWARDS YOURSELF

This is powerful. You may be able to relate to it. Trying to escape the body you are in right now may feel like a prison sentence, and every time you feel like you are about to break free, you are right back where you first started, unhappy and trapped in the prison cell.

But there is a proven route and you will escape as long as you follow it. Cut out the things that prevent you from losing fat and make you go back to the start, like chocolate, alcohol, not exercising, excuses, and then add the things you need to (like exercise) and you will be free. But you just can't do it, your mindset is not strong enough.

> ## ✓ TOP TIP mindset
>
> Get in the habit of finishing everything you start, even if you don't like it. For example, if you read a book or watch a film and then, halfway through it, you don't like it, make sure you finish it, because when you do things like exercise or nutrition, I can guarantee that you are going to hit times where you will just want to give up or finish earlier than planned. For example, if you are working out on a running machine and you only have 5 minutes left, your mind will say 'just stop'. However, if you get into a habit of finishing everything you start, it will become useful for those times when you will want to quit a few minutes early or finish a nutrition plan a couple of days too soon etc.

# • MINDSET TASK 1 •

### Step 1

I want you to think of someone you love more than anyone else in the world! It could be your mother, father, son, daughter, best friend or even a pet. It must be someone that you would do anything in the world for.

### Step 2

Okay, now I want you to take a minute and think about why you love this person or animal so much. Think about all the good times you have had together. Before you read on make sure you think about this person or animal.

### Step 3

Now imagine that person is your child, who is trapped in a prison and cannot escape. You can see them through a camera and they are so scared it breaks your heart to see them like this.

However, you have a proven route to help them escape this prison sentence and you have full control of what they do.

On this route, they are not allowed to eat any chocolate, sweets, fast food, or drink any alcohol, and must exercise three times a week for 12 months. If they do, they will never escape and your child will never be as happy as you would like. Remember, this is in your control entirely, you decide if they have the treats or if they workout or not.

Would you make sure they did what they needed to do or would you allow them to have the odd treat and miss the odd exercise knowing that they will be trapped there for the rest of their lives?

I'm guessing you would make sure they followed the proven route.

If you would do that for your child (or the person you love), why wouldn't you do it for yourself?

## THE 4 ELEMENTS OF MINDSET

To help get into the right mindset there are 4 elements to consider:

1. Goals

2. Vision

3. Barriers

4. Achieve

They all work together like a team. When you have the right **goals** and **vision** you will overcome the **barriers** and **achieve.**

Let's go back to that holiday. Their **goal** was to go on holiday. Their **vision** was whether they were going to be wearing a bikini or snow boots and why. The barriers were the cost of the holiday, what they needed to buy, when they could go and for how long. The difference between a holiday and trying to lose fat is that a holiday is external from your normal day-to-day life and losing fat is internal within your normal day-to-day life.

If you want to break free from an unhealthy, overweight body and never go back you have to change your lifestyle and understand it is going to be a change you make forever! Not just a couple of weeks.

With a holiday, you subconsciously know your life will be completely different for a week or so. Instead of waking up and going to work, you sunbathe by a pool or climb a mountain to ski down the other side.

For the period you are on holiday your lifestyle changes and you can get away with things that you can't do at home. For instance, not working and not having to take your kids to school, drinking cocktails every day etc. Once your holiday is finished you go back to your original lifestyle.

When you are trying to break free from obesity, this will not be the case, you will have to focus on changing your lifestyle forever. It's not just 2 weeks, 3 months or 6 months but for the rest of your life. You must learn to change your habits from bad to good. Otherwise, if you don't, your bad habit will always push you back and stop you from fully escaping the unhealthy, overweight body you are not happy with.

A GOAL TELLS YOUR MIND WHICH
WAY YOU ARE GOING. WITHOUT A
GOAL, YOU ARE GUESSING WHERE
TO GO AND, THEREFORE, YOUR
MIND GETS CONFUSED. GOALS HELP
TO GIVE YOUR MINDSET CLARITY.

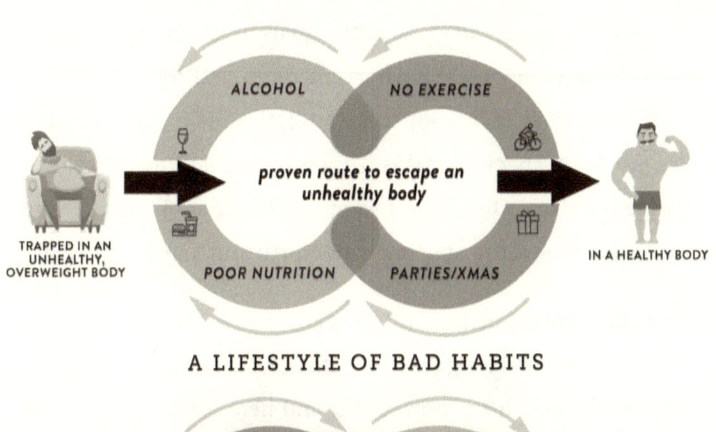


A LIFESTYLE OF BAD HABITS



A LIFESTYLE OF GOOD HABITS

To get in the right mindset you need to consciously break down your **Goals, Visions, Barriers** and **Achievements**. I have created tasks for you so that by the end of this chapter, you are going to be laser-focused on what you want to achieve and why. Do not skip to the end because it is important to understand the rest of this mindset before you go to the questions.

## Goals

A **goal** tells your mind which way you are going. Without a goal, you are guessing where to go and, therefore, your mind gets confused. Goals help to give your mindset clarity.

It's very good to have specific goals and always good to have more than one (e.g. short, medium and long term). An unspecific goal is 'I want to lose weight' or 'I want to travel the world'. A specific goal is 'I want to lose 112lbs (51kg) and go from a size 22 to 12' or 'I want to visit 5 out of 7 of the continents of the world, starting with North and South America'.

You then break them down into short (6-12 weeks) medium (3-6 months) and long (6-12 months). Others will do it slightly differently, but this is how I do it and here are some examples of specific goals.

## Goal examples

Short term: I want to lose 42lbs (19kg) within 3 months and drop 3 dress sizes.

Medium: To lose 70lbs (32kg) within 6 months and be at least a size 14.

Long: To lose 112lbs (51kg) and be a size 12 before going down to a size 10.

This is just an example. When you are on a fat-loss journey, it's very important to look at the longer-term picture and add the physical goals that you want to achieve. Because if you do not have longer-term goals in place when you have achieved the dress size you are after, you'll have nothing else to stay focused on.

Personally, I would recommend creating physical goals over appearance goals – such as completing a half marathon, obstacle course, or maybe even a triathlon. These work best because you must train for all these events, otherwise you will struggle. The bonus is that, as you train for these events, your appearance will improve.

## CASE STUDY: EMMA

*Emma was a size 20 when we met. When we discussed her goals, Emma told me she could only dream about being a size 16 and that reaching this size would change her life. She wasn't interested in the short or medium-term goals; she just had the finish line in sight.*

*I worked with Emma for a few months and even though I saw she was happier for being healthier and fitter, she was so focused on the end result of being a size 16 she disregarded all the little wins that she achieved along the way.*

*When she achieved her dream goal of being a size 16, Emma didn't even stop to celebrate. She just set a new goal of becoming a size 12. Emma had completely forgotten that she'd previously thought being a size 16 would make her really happy.*

In order to understand how far you have come, it's very important to celebrate the wins along the way.

# Vision

A **Vision** is a clearly defined picture of your future that gives you purpose. It will help you to understand why you are trying to achieve a certain goal and attach the right emotions to your journey. This, in turn, will give you the motivation to succeed. If you are trying to lose fat, you are not just doing it for fun, there will always be a bigger reason why you want to do this.

A lot of times people will cover up the real reason because they don't believe they can actually achieve it. Some people will say they need to lose weight because they are too heavy. This is a great reason, but the real reason could be that they are sick of being the biggest one in their group of friends, or upset that they can't go shopping because they know they are too big for the clothes in certain shops. Or they no longer have sex with their partners because they are too embarrassed with the way they look and will only do it with the lights off. These are only a couple of reasons and if you are reading this trying to escape your body, then I bet you can relate to them.

Once you are true to yourself and truly understand the real reason why you want to lose fat, this will then become your vision.

## Vision example

'I want to lose weight so that I can feel sexy for my husband like I used to.'

That is only one sentence, so when you write it out you want to make it as detailed as possible. The more information the better.

## Step 1

Take your time to write this down on a piece of paper. I just want to warn you that this might feel quite emotional; so you may need to take a minute afterwards.

1. On a scale of 1-10, how much do you want to change? 1 is not very and 10 is the most important thing in the world to you right now.

2. How long have you been trying to change?

3. How is it affecting your life? (Be honest here and take the time to write down how it is affecting you in every way)

4. Who else is it affecting? (e.G. your kids because you can't do as much as you would like to)

5. Is there anything you don't do because of the position you're in? (For example, you don't go shopping or go out due to your lack of confidence, and be honest here)

6. Write down why you don't do the things you've listed in each of the answers to question 5 above.

7. How does it make you feel that you are not doing those things?

8. How will it make you feel if you still haven't changed a year from now?

9. I'm going to ask you again, on a scale of 1-10, how much do you want to change? 1 is not very and 10 is the most important thing to you right now.

## Step 2

I want you to put yourself in fantasy mode now, so don't think about what is achievable when you're answering these questions. Instead, think about what you dream of. Ready?

1. If you stood in front of a mirror and looked back at yourself, what would you see that would make you smile from one side of your face to the other? Define it right down to the style and the colour of everything that you are wearing and the occasion you are dressed for. (E.g. you're wearing a red polka dot dress and ready to go to a ball with your husband)

2. If that really happened, how would it make you feel?

3. What physical challenge do you dream of achieving. (E.g. running the London marathon, climbing a mountain)

4. How would the knowledge that you could complete it make you feel?

5. Who would notice it and who would be the proudest of you when you did achieve these goals?

### Step 3

I want you to write down this vision you have just created. I want you to write it as a story on a big piece of paper (e.g. it's September 2020 and I am celebrating climbing a mountain earlier that day. I am in a size 10 red dress at a very fancy restaurant with my husband and I can see how proud he is of me etc. Go into as much detail as possible). Once you have written your vision, I want you to read it back to yourself and highlight the best bit. I then want you to put your vision somewhere you can see it every day, e.g. on the fridge or your desk at work.

### Step 4

Now, write down when you would like to start your journey to achieve these goals?

## Barriers

**Barriers** are anything that could prevent you from breaking free from your unhealthy, overweight body. This could be: money, time, work, kids, addictions, bad habits, knowledge, emotions and hormones, partners, holidays, festivals… The list goes on. You need to be aware of the barriers you face so that you can strengthen your mindset and not give in to them.

I have worked with a lot of people and what I call barriers, others will call excuses. It is very frustrating and saddening that people keep using barriers as excuses when I try to help them. Giving up your goal because of one setback is like slashing your other three tires because one is flat.

I am not going to go into all of them, but let's use one of the most common: money. This is the worst excuse and one that really upsets me.

*Barrier example:*

"I can't afford to lose weight."

They will say they can't afford to join a gym or get any form of coaching. Yet they have a car on finance, are out partying each weekend, need to buy a new outfit for each weekend or enjoy annual holidays. They want to get a tattoo or they "need" to have an allowance for make-up each month or coffees and snacks at their local café.

If you are sitting there and thinking, "I don't do any of that," and you still can't afford to lose weight, this is also just a barrier. There is endless free information on the internet and the only thing it will cost you is your time, as you will have to spend a few months on researching and testing what works best for you.

These sort of people opt-in for free weight-loss challenges or courses put on by professionals to show people that they know what they are talking about. Then, within the weight-loss challenge (which is a try before you buy kinda thing) they will gain great results quickly for free. So far, so good. Then, when the challenge comes to an end and they have an opportunity to participate in a life-changing programme which costs money they will opt-out and go back to their original lives instead, and continue to wonder how to lose weight and then just repeat the cycle.

This reason is very frustrating because you can see they are in pain but they will not do the things that are required to make their lives better. Instead, they allow these (excuses) barriers to get in the way and just settle for an unhappy life.

If you are trapped in a body that makes you depressed, anxious, knocks your confidence etc. and someone is offering you a course that is going to change your life, then do it! It's worth more than any holiday, car, jewellery, make-up and your beloved cups of coffee combined. As soon as you start realising that breaking free is the most important thing, you will start figuring out how to overcome other barriers.

## • MINDSET TASK 3 •

Rate your level of happiness right now, 10 being extremely happy and on cloud 9 and 1 hating life and wanting it to be over. Okay, if you scored lower than a 6 for whatever reason, ask yourself this question before making any decision in life: is this going to take me closer to a 10? Or 1? Everything that you do should be purely about making you happier until you are scoring over 8.

This task aims to figure out all the barriers that might be in your way and then create a solution.

## Step 1

Take the time to fill out the table below. On one side of it put all your barriers and on the other create all the solutions. At the end of this chapter, I will send you to a place where you can do the mindset challenge that I have created. (I have created templates you can print off.)

| Problems/Barriers/Excuses | Solution |
|---|---|
| Time | I will wake up at 5am to workout during the week. I will cook all my food that I need to eat throughout the week on Sunday. |
| Son's birthday party | Instead of unhealthy snacks, I'm going to find healthy recipes, for example, healthy brownies that taste like brownies. |
| Friend's birthday | I will take them out for a healthy lunch and not go to the birthday party as they will have another one next year. |

## Step 2

Always ask yourself this question whenever you are about to do something: is this going to help me get closer to a 10 or closer to a 1?

You don't want something like this to happen. It's Friday, you have just finished work and you are around a 5 on the happy scale of life. Everyone you know is going out for drinks and a little party, and you know that if you go it's going to be great, but you will probably stay out all night, be hungover in the morning and feel closer to a 3, but you do it anyway, to drown your sorrows and celebrate the end of the week.

The next morning you wake up feeling like crap, and you realise how much money you have spent and it will take you a few days to get back to a 4.

It's now the following Tuesday and you are feeling fat so you go to an exercise class and get back to a 5 on the happy scale of life.

Then your friends invite you out for a meal with them and a bottle of wine or a few beers whilst you chit-chat. You have a great night but you are back to a 3 when you wake up because you have consumed lots of things that will prevent you from losing fat. This cycle continues and you never really get any closer to where you want to be on the happy scale of life.

## Achieve

You **achieve** when you successfully reach your goal through effort, skill, and courage. This is the final piece of the mindset puzzle. Once you have the other three in place all you have to do is find out how you are going to achieve your goal. This sounds simple, but it's not easy.

This is the part where you may need to reach out to someone to help you create a proven route to help you escape an unhealthy body and break down exactly how you are going to **Achieve** your **Goal.**

If you are going through your fat-loss journey and feel like you are going off-track, come back to these 4 elements and go through this again. It will help you refocus on what you want.

I have created a mindset challenge which breaks these elements down and you can do it for free. Visit **www.chrismarcoflores. com** to take the challenge.

## YOU WILL NEED TO FIND WILL

Who is WILL? WILL stands for WILLPOWER!

Now, what is willpower? It is the control exerted to do something or restrain impulses. Turning down a cigarette or chocolate cake, saying no to a Chinese takeaway and having chicken and salad instead, or going to the gym when you want to go to sleep takes willpower. It is closely linked with mindset because the stronger your mindset, the more certain you are of what you are trying to achieve and why, the stronger your WILL will be.

The difference between mindset and WILL is that your mindset gets you in the right state of mind to do something. Your WILL is used to actually do it.

For example, it's a Sunday and you get yourself into a mindset to workout the following Monday morning before work at 6am. When Monday morning 6am comes along and you wake up tired, it's your WILLPOWER that makes you get out of bed and workout.

As I explained about the mind, WILL is like a muscle. The more you train the stronger it gets. It's very important to have a strong WILL when it comes to breaking bad habits and creating new ones, like instead of going straight home after work and watching TV, going straight to the gym.

A great method is to learn to say no to bad temptation and substitute it for something good. Look at something you may like, say no and replace it with something healthy. So instead of a chocolate bar have a handful of nuts. It is an incredibly powerful method.

At first, the handful of nuts or piece of fruit will not satisfy you at all because your body knows the satisfaction it receives when eating chocolate (or whatever your temptation is) and it will be expecting the same level of satisfaction. When you eat something else, like nuts or a bit of fruit, your body and mind will tell you: this is not what I expect, give me what I'm used to.

If you successfully say no and choose something else, you are strengthening your WILL every day, so it will become easier in the future. Not only will you start to feel stronger and more satisfied, you will start feeling the benefit of having something good over something bad.

## ✓ TOP TIPS on how to grow WILL

### 1. Make yourself a plan and stick to it

This can be any kind of plan, but here you are trying to escape an unhealthy, overweight body. Get a nutrition and exercise plan and force yourself to stick to it. Even if it doesn't fit in with your lifestyle, make it work. This is how I learnt best with all my personal training experience. I used to buy other personal trainers plans from around the world and stick to them and not only would I get results but I would learn from them.

### 2. Get more sleep

I bet some of you who are reading this will thank me for this tip! Getting a good night's sleep between 6.5-9 hours (some athletes will try to sleep for 10) will decrease your stress levels and help you become more focused.

THE DIFFERENCE BETWEEN
MINDSET AND WILL IS THAT YOUR
MINDSET GETS YOU IN THE RIGHT
STATE OF MIND TO DO SOMETHING.
YOUR WILL IS USED TO
ACTUALLY DO IT.

However, I am slightly contradicting myself here because as my clients get stronger, I encourage them to spend 2-4 weeks pushing the mind by waking up a lot earlier than they could imagine. This is to show them that you don't have to live a systematic lifestyle. Don't worry about that just yet.

## 3. Replenish the body (others like to call it meditating)

I have never really been one for meditating in the fashionable way of sitting down, legs crossed, thumb to finger, and humming away, because I have never been taught how to do it or given it enough time to feel the real benefits. What I do and thoroughly love is something I call an undesignated run or walk.

You set aside a **minimum** of 1 hour once a week and just walk or run by yourself, preferably somewhere with nice views to clear your head. There is no destination, because you walk or run until you feel satisfied, then turn back. This will take you out of your world. It is the best de-stress mechanism you could ever have. If you suffer from depression, you need to learn this method as quickly as you can. I like to walk or run to music, but you could just listen to nature. I know I said it is preferable to do it with a nice view, but you can do it anywhere, even if you are in a crowded city. I discovered this method by mistake in London.

## 4. Exercise

There are two different types of exercise.

You can exercise gently without raising your heart rate at all, which is great for your health and good for recovery.

You can elevate your heart rate, which can be quite uncomfortable although it does come with a list of great benefits. You should try and raise your heart rate at least 3 times a week. (I will go into more depth later in this book.)

It takes a lot of WILLpower to continue when you feel uncomfortable, and pushing yourself through exercising is the best way to increase it.

## 5. Learning to say NO

It is so easy to give in to temptation and peer pressure, whether it be a work colleague trying to get you to eat a chocolate biscuit with them or your friends trying to persuade you to join them on a night out. If you are always someone who says yes, you will need the willpower to say NO. When you start to say NO, you will feel proud of yourself and strengthen your WILL.

# MY STORY: DE-STRESSING SAVED MY LIFE

After the US Army, I went on a working holiday trip to Ayia Napa in Cyprus and I spent 3 months drinking every day there without a care in a world. Then the summer came to an end, the fun stopped and I moved to London to find a job.

It had been a whirlwind, from being in the Army where I jumped out of planes and went on combat missions every day, to an unbelievable party holiday in Cyprus, to becoming an estate agent in London. As you could imagine I found it very hard to adapt. I had a very bad spell of depression. I was not enjoying life.

There was one day I will never forget. I came home from work and my housemate said if I didn't give him £200 towards the rent, even though it wasn't due until the beginning of the month, he was going to kick me out. I didn't have the money and I didn't know what to do. As you can imagine, I didn't sleep all night, my emotions were going crazy and it felt like I could explode.

I was in Hammersmith and I was so stressed in the morning, I had to get out of the flat to try and clear my head. So I put my headphones in and just started walking in any direction. I had no clue where I was going, but I was trying to figure out what I was going to do. I must have walked for 3 hours. I stopped to have a bit of lunch (Nando's) by myself and continued to walk.

After 5 hours of non-stop walking, it suddenly felt like I had a moment of euphoria.

One big rush of joy and happiness went right through my body and all my stress was gone. I didn't have one bit of depression left in my body, and it was all from that one walk. My body released so many endorphins that it completely changed me. It also gave me a lot of clarity on what I wanted and needed to do with my life. I paid what my housemate asked for and made it my priority to change the situation I was in.

I realised I was in an environment (the flat) where there was unnecessary negativity. So I sucked it up, rang my dad and asked if I could come home for a short while to help sort myself out.

Secondly, I was doing something that I felt like I had to do and did not enjoy it. I loved fitness and everything to do with health and fitness. That was when I decided I finally wanted to find a career within fitness.

Then, every week, I would dedicate a bit of time to go for a similar walk. An hour would be more than enough as I was doing this so regularly. Although the longer I would leave it, the longer I would have to go for a walk.

You're probably wondering how going for a head-clearing walk or run can grow the power of your WILL. By forcing yourself to meditate or go for an undesignated walk or run twice a week, and committing to sticking to that plan, you will be developing your will and doing something good for yourself. Double win.

Everyone meditates differently. Find your way of meditation and have the willpower to keep it up.

## BREAK THE MINDSET MOULD

Even a fraction of a change to our lives can unsettle us, so it is a very good idea to learn to get out of a systematic lifestyle.

To some people, it is not normal to wake up before 6am and workout. Mark Wahlberg is known for waking up at 4am to workout before a day's work. He is in incredible shape because he puts the work in.

Or you might be someone who wakes up before 6am but goes to bed very early, so doing anything in the evening is off-limits, especially exercise.

Triple H from WWE is known for doing midnight workouts to make sure he stays in shape.

Now, these are some extreme examples. But you should look at them as an inspiration. Sometimes, you have to do something out of the ordinary to be able to accomplish things that may seem impossible.

Learn to break the system and your mind will begin to open.

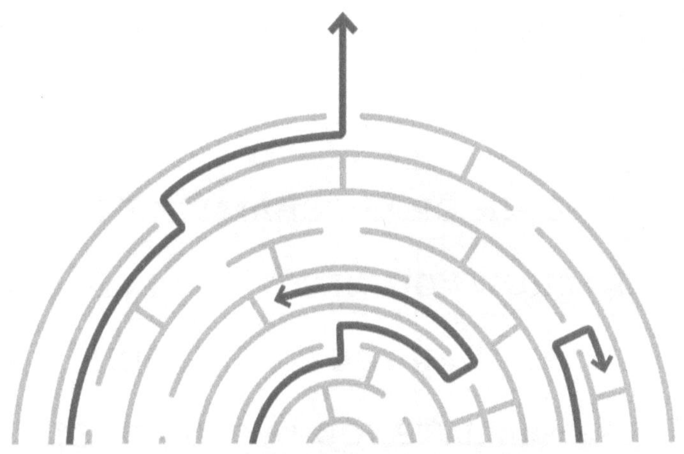

# VITAL ACTIVITY 2
## Challenge

## WHAT IS A CHALLENGE?

Challenges are the best way to measure your fitness and push your mind further than you could imagine, to turn the Impossible into the Possible. On this journey, you will face mini-challenges every day. Challenges are a chance to test your mindset.

Sticking to a meal plan is going to be a mental challenge. Making yourself do fitness sessions is going to be a mental and physical

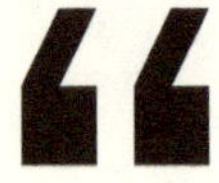

THE AIM OF ANY CHALLENGE IS
TO SHOW YOU THAT YOU CAN DO
MORE THAN YOU CAN IMAGINE,
ESPECIALLY IF YOU TAKE ON ONES
YOU FEEL YOU CANNOT COMPLETE.

challenge. Learning to increase your fitness intensity is going to be a mental and physical challenge. Not giving in to temptation is going to be a mental challenge. And that is just to name a few.

The aim of any challenge is to show you that you can do more than you can imagine, especially if you take on ones you feel you cannot complete.

## WHY ARE CHALLENGES A VITAL ACTIVITY?

Challenges are by far my most favourite part of this and one of the most important elements. They push you outside your comfort zone, show you what you can achieve and give you a huge sense of satisfaction.

As people get into fitness, they get the "fitness bug" and for a period of their life, they cannot get enough fitness. This is the position you want to try and get yourself into. But if people train just to train with no real purpose and have no real focus as to why they are doing so, the fitness bug will sooner or later die out.

I know this because it has happened to me, and before I knew it, my fitness levels dropped and I had put on more weight than I thought I ever would.

The people who stay with fitness are the ones who are always challenging themselves. People who have a reason to be fit.

Imagine if you had two people and one was training for a triathlon race that was in 5 weeks' time and the other was just going to the gym just to train. Who do you think is going to be the more focused? Of course, the person training for a triathlon because he knows why he is training and, if he is smart enough, will have a structured plan to follow.

If you are escaping an unhealthy body, it is very important to put challenges in place because it will help you to remain focused.

You should be challenging yourself right from the beginning, and give yourself a new challenge at least every 2 months. When you have finished one challenge you should be already setting up the next, so you will always have something to aim for.

## WHAT HAPPENS IF YOU DON'T SET YOURSELF THE RIGHT CHALLENGE?

If you don't focus your energy around a challenge, you are unlikely to see any real results because you have no goal to strive for, and can't tell if you've achieved it or not.

If you focus on the wrong challenge, your focus can be in the wrong place, and when that happens, you will never achieve what you desire. For example, when people are looking to achieve long-term fat loss so they can be fitter, healthier, happier and more comfortable in their body, they focus too much on trying to lose weight when, in fact, they should be focusing more on changing their lifestyle. They need to become fitter, healthier and completely ignore the scales.

Remember you are trying to change your lifestyle, not just your diet.

You should focus more on things like running one mile and then turning that one mile into two miles and then three miles, or a different type of fitness if you don't want to run, rather than just focusing on how much you weigh.

Your main challenge is to become fitter and healthier; when you achieve this your fat-loss will follow. Train your mind to focus on becoming fitter, rather than focus on the numbers on the scales.

## BIG CHALLENGES GET BIG RESULTS

The challenges I am talking about here are those that scare you or you think are impossible. These challenges push you way out of your comfort zone into a whole new world. If you fear a challenge and think you cannot do it, it will make you stronger when you do complete it, physically and mentally.

Do not wait until you think you are ready for the challenge. By all means train for it, but completing a challenge you do not feel ready for will make you stronger than completing a challenge that you have fully trained for.

## IF IT FRIGHTENS YOU, IT'S A CHALLENGE

What kind of challenges should you do? When should they be done? Why should you fear the challenge? How many should you do?

There is a level of exercise called 'Fear the session'. Every single challenge should be like this.

That doesn't mean to say you shouldn't do a 5k run because it doesn't frighten you; by all means, do as many challenges as you can. But every 6 weeks you want to have a challenge that is going to really frighten you.

This doesn't have to continue for the rest of your life, it is just needed whilst you are escaping an unhealthy body (although you may get hooked on challenges). Having something like this in place will help you to change your lifestyle as it will help you stay consistently focused.

Challenges can be anything you desire, but they must physically place some kind of demand on your body. Don't just do the challenges by yourself because you won't have any real accountability.

I don't mean sign up for an event with your best friend, sign up instead to an event where there will be others participating and cheering you on (even if you do not know the other participants). There are thousands of challenges that companies put on throughout the year, such as an obstacle course, 5k race, marathon, Iron man and triathlon. Anything to do with physical activity is acceptable.

Yes! It might cost you some money to enter a challenge that is going to push your mind mentally (although there are plenty around £30-£50), but that is much better than wasting the money on cocktails all night which will destroy your body.

# • CHALLENGE TASK 1 •

## Step 1

I'm going to list 10 different challenges.

1. Run 1 mile

2. Run a 5k race

3. Complete a triathlon (Super sprint – 200m swim, 12-mile bike ride and 2.5-mile run)

4. Complete a 10k obstacle course

5. Complete a triathlon (Sprint – 400m swim, 12.4-mile bike ride, 3.1-mile run)

6. Run a half marathon (13.1-mile run)

7. Fight in a boxing match

8. Run a marathon (26.2-mile run)

9. Complete a triathlon (Olympic – 1-mile swim, 20-mile bike ride and 6-mile run)

10. Finish an Iron man

Did you feel any fear when you imagined doing any of these challenges? If the answer is yes, it is a good sign.

## Step 2

I want you to pick a challenge that you think you cannot complete. Now, if you have never run in your life or find running very hard, pick a 1mile run or maybe even a 5km run. Don't pick a marathon.

## Step 3

I want you to finish the rest of the chapter and then, once you have picked a challenge, go on the internet, find an event within the next 6 weeks and sign up for it. For example, if it is a 10k obstacle course, type into Google "10k obstacle courses". You will have hundreds to choose from. You may have to travel to do the event, but I promise you it will be worth it.

## Step 4

Prepare to complete this event within the next 6 weeks. You might have to reach out to someone who can give you a training plan to help.

---

### ✓ TOP TIP

If you wait for family, friends or a colleague to be ready to do a challenge alongside you, because you are too scared to complete the event alone, you may never end up doing it. Don't wait for others to join you. Sign up for it and if others follow then that is a bonus.

# CASE STUDY: LYNN

*Before I go into this case study, I said I would help you to understand the importance of each mission. The case study I am about to share will explain the power of the first mission, 'unlock'.*

*The aim of unlock is to help you realise you are capable of more than you think you are and how this will then create a snowball effect.*

*Lynn was another great client who has now become a good friend of mine. When we first met, her only aim was to lose weight, 28lbs (13kg) to be exact. When we first spoke, I asked her briefly if she would like to do a 10k obstacle course. Her reply was, "Maybe after a year's worth of training."*

*I didn't say anything else. I got her past the first level of exercising which was 'Ease yourself in'. (I will explain the levels of exercise later in this book.) It only took a week for Lynn to get past this level. The following week, I pulled Lynn aside and told her that there was a 10k obstacle event coming up in 5 weeks' time and she needed to sign up.*

*She still insisted that she would do it in a year's time. I then told her the reason why I wanted her to do it. I didn't want it to be easy for her. I wanted her to struggle at the event to show her that it was possible and to get rid of that fear in her head and to 'unlock' her mind.*

*After a little encouragement, Lynn finally agreed. She was far from happy but I didn't care (not because I am heartless, but because I knew what it was going to do for her).*

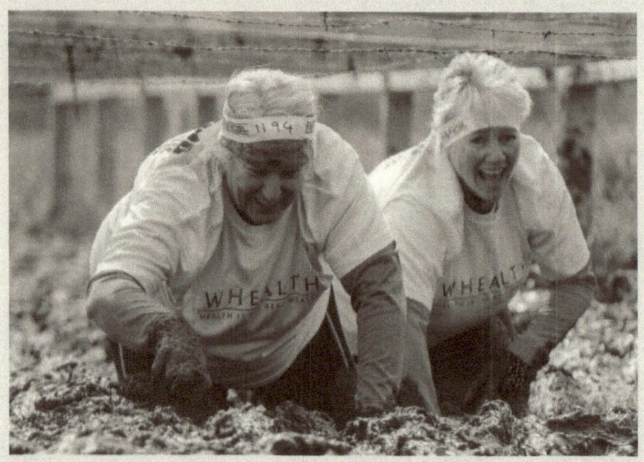

*Then, 6 weeks on from when we'd first met, we stood at the start line of the 10k obstacle course. I had most of my clients there, full of fear and anxiety, worrying that they wouldn't complete it! Everyone else in the event was clearly fitter than any of my clients, and it was a tough race. Even though we were the slowest and last group to finish, in my mind, we were the biggest winners! By a long shot! And I was more than proud of every single one of them.*

*This challenge unlocked Lynn's mind and since then she has completed another 10k obstacle course, climbed Ben Nevis and signed up to a half marathon, all within the same year. I only asked her to do the first one, all the others were off her*

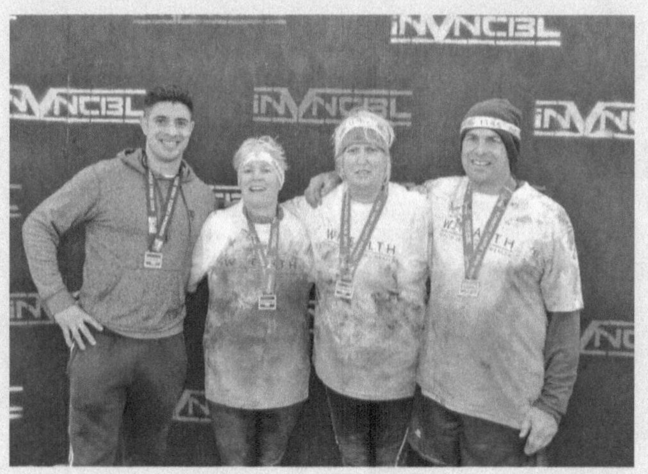

## MY STORY: BASIC TRAINING

My British Army Basic Training lasted for 26 weeks. Fifty-five people started the course and the first 6 weeks involved physical training every day. I'm pretty sure this was to get rid of the ones who couldn't stick to it. After the first 6 weeks, over half of the men had quit. After the first 6 weeks had finished, one of the sergeants would put a piece of paper on our noticeboard at the beginning of each week, telling us what we would be doing in the upcoming week.

I remember when I first saw it. (Remember, we'd had 6 weeks' worth of training, so we were fitter than when we first arrived.)

IT DOESN'T HAPPEN OVERNIGHT.
IT TAKES MORE THAN ONE
CHALLENGE TO BREAK
THROUGH AN UNHEALTHY BODY.

It said: Week 7, Monday – 3-mile run; Wednesday circuit training; Friday 2-mile ruck march with 5lbs (2kg) in your bags.

It scared me because I wasn't mentally strong enough to think I could complete the challenges.

Each week it got tougher because the miles and weight increased. By the 16th week, the sheet on the wall said: Week 16, Monday, 6-mile run and Wednesday, 6-mile ruck march with 25lbs (11kg) in our bags and again it scared me because I wasn't mentally tough enough at the time to complete it.

By week 16, I would have been jumping for joy if I had seen Week 16, Monday 2-mile run and Wednesday 2-mile ruck march with 5lbs (2kg) in your bags, because my mind would have thought it was a walk in the park.

At first, the challenges scared me. That was until I completed them. Even though I thought I couldn't do them, it **unlocked** my mind every time.

After completing so many frightening challenges you reach a point where something switches in your head. You have proven to yourself you can do so much more than your body tells you and so you become fearless about any challenge that comes your way.

I like to call this the military mindset. (However, you do not have to be in the military to gain this mindset.) The first 6 months of my journey through the Army was the hardest

6 months of my whole life but was also the most rewarding journey of my life! This journey is most likely going to be the toughest of your life, but it will also be the most rewarding one that will change your life forever!

## CASE STUDY: ROSIE

*Rosie is another great client. She was a size 22 when I first met her. She had tried all the diets under the sun and created a big bad habit, which had become a life pattern. She would start a diet, lose a lot of weight and reach the first level on the mountain, and would then slowly go back to her original lifestyle that kept her in the unhealthy, overweight body she didn't like being in. Of course, this meant that she never got to the top, and always ended back at square one, at the bottom of the mountain, looking for a new diet. She thought it was going to be physically impossible for her to change.*

*She also told me she couldn't even think about walking a mile as her fitness level was so poor. She signed up to my programme* **The Weight is Over**. *I also encouraged her to do a 10k obstacle course within the first 6 weeks. (The same one that Lynn did.)*

*Within 6 weeks Rosie had completed the obstacle course, but it didn't give her the feeling she'd hoped for. She was expecting a moment of joy, but because it was so tough, Rosie didn't have the energy to think about celebrating. Personally, I think she was happy that it was just over.*

*The challenge **'unlocked'** her mind because she was able to see that she was capable of doing it. However, it still didn't change her mindset completely the way I needed it too. That is why you have to have more than just one challenge to get to that military mindset.*

*After 12 weeks she lost 4 dress sizes and 42lbs (19kg)! That was when she hit the 4th phase and felt the joy. It was the first time she thought it was possible for her to escape the body she despised being in.*

It doesn't happen overnight. It takes more than one challenge to break through an unhealthy overweight body.

Anything is possible. If you want something bad enough, follow these principles long enough and you will achieve it.

## SHALLOW HAL WILL SWALLOW YOU UP

Is getting out of an unhealthy, overweight body a mental or physical challenge? And what is Shallow Hal? I like to use the term 'Shallow Hal', which is inspired by the film *Shallow Hal*, starring Jack Black.

If you don't know the movie, at the beginning Hal was a very shallow person who didn't have any respect for anyone and judged them on the way they looked. He then bumps into a guy who hypnotises him to only see the beauty in people. As you can imagine, his perspective completely shifts.

From my experience, all of my clients who start off overweight feel 'fat'. When they lose a noticeable amount of weight, they can see progress. However, they mentally still feel like the person when they first started, overweight and 'fat'. So I need to create a solution to make sure that they can get out of this mindset and understand what they have achieved.

But before I talk about that, you must understand that a lot of people who go through a fat-loss journey, neglect the small wins along the way. Then, when they reach their big goal, it doesn't feel like the achievement they were hoping for. Remember Emma, who was desperate to be a size 16 but then when she got there, decided she would be happier if she was a size 12. She is not alone.

There are two reasons for this.

1.  They are in a Shallow Hal mindset and still feel like the person they were when they first started their journey.

2.  They don't appreciate the wins along the way.

You must actively get out of this mindset! If you do not, you will remain just as unhappy as when you first started, regardless of your results.

There are two proven ways that work wonders.

1. **Find someone to help**: As soon as you have reached your first milestone, e.g. losing 14lbs (6kg), dropping 1 dress size or running 1 mile for the first time, find someone who is in the same position you were when you first started and teach them to do what you have done. Every time you hit another milestone find another person who is where you were when you first started.

   Doing this will psychologically help you to realise where you once were and how far you have come. You'll see that you are not that person anymore. This will also help you to enjoy the journey and not the results.

2. **If you cannot find anyone to help:** Challenges are incredible for making you realise how far you can push your mind, and by doing them frequently, it will help you understand how far you have come and enable you to break free from the Shallow Hal mindset.

## CASE STUDY: ANDREW

*My client Andrew is a perfect example. I spoke about him previously to show you what he was able to achieve, but let's dig deeper and find out what was going on inside his head and how he overcame it. When I first met Andrew, he had already lost 70lbs (32kg) but was worried about putting it back on, as he had done before. During the first consultation, I did a little digging and found out Andrew wanted to go to his work's Christmas party, which he had never been able to attend due to his lack of confidence. So, I helped him to create a vision and got him to imagine what it would feel like to be at his Christmas party. I also asked him, if I had a magic wand, what would he like to be wearing at this party. He told me he had always worn baggy clothes to hide his body but would love to wear a fitted white medium-sized shirt.*

*So, before we got started, I told him to go and buy a white medium shirt and keep it in view so that he was able to see it every day.*

*We went through the programme and Andrew ended up losing 56 more pounds, a total of 126lb (57kg), and he had to go and buy a small shirt because the medium was too big.*

*His fitness levels went through the roof, and he started doing things he had never done before, like push-ups and pull-ups.*

*Amazing, right?! That's what I thought. But because Andrew had been a big man all his life, he still felt like the person he once was, so he still felt worthless. His confidence had been knocked, and he still wasn't in the place he wanted to be.*

*So, I encouraged him to sign up for a challenge. A 10k obstacle course called 'Mission unbreakable' (the same one that I convinced Lynn and Rosie to do).*

*He didn't want to do it because he had become very anxious and had no confidence, and this would be a very public challenge.*

*I managed to get him to sign up but he would tell me why he couldn't do it every week up until the challenge.*

*"I have to work."*

*"My neighbours' dog has died."*

*"It's not the right time."*

*"I'll do it next time."*

*The excuses were endless.*

*But I wouldn't let him off the hook! Even on the day itself, I had to make sure he turned up.*

*There were 11 of us in our group on this challenge and most of them were "fighting the fear", as they were all worried that they wouldn't be able to complete it, including Andrew.*

*The thing is, I knew Andrew would fly around the course as he was a lot fitter than he realised.*

*We were at the race and in the queue for our group to run and you could see the anticipation on his face. You could just tell he wanted to turn around and go home, but within 2 minutes of the race beginning, Andrew was a different man! He flew around that course, like I knew he would.*

*Within the first 10 minutes, Andrew realised how far he had come and throughout the race, he was helping the others*

## THE DIFFERENT TYPES OF CHALLENGES

I like to define challenges as things that push you out of the comfort zone that you know, and will reward you once you have completed them.

You could do a challenge and the reward might be something physical, like you might have completed a challenge to win something. Then there are other challenges where you do not receive anything physical, but you are rewarded with a feeling inside that money cannot buy. These rewards help you to grow as a person and learn about yourself. Personally, I think these are by far the best rewards.

There are TV shows that I can use to prove this.

The first challenge that I mentioned, where people win something tangible are shows like *Who Wants to Be a Millionaire*, where they win life-changing money for answering questions or even shows like *Fear Factor*, an old US show where contestants won life-changing money for succeeding in 3 physical and mental challenges. Of course, the winners felt completely over the moon about the amazing reward.

A great TV show that demonstrates the second challenge, where the reward is you grow as a person, is *Who Dares Wins*. If you have never seen the show before, ex-British Special Forces service members get 20 ordinary working civilians with no connection to the military lifestyle and put them through challenges to give them a little taste of what it is like to be able to pass a selection process to be accepted into the British Special Forces.

In 7 days or so (the time is not revealed) the contestants are pushed to their physical and mental limits. They have the options to leave at any time and only a few people finish. Every time someone quits they are interviewed and you can see that even the people who do not make it until the end have been broken down to the point where it opens their minds. They are amazed that they have achieved things they would never have thought were possible and, within a few short days, have changed for the better, due to earning the rewarding feeling of growth.

If you would like to experience that feeling of growth yourself, which I personally seek at least twice a year, you need to take on a challenge that is beyond your limits.

Like I said before, if you think you can walk/run 1 mile, go and sign up for a 5k race, or if you struggle to think about completing a 5k race, sign up to a 10k race. (Not a marathon as it is too far beyond your reach.) However, if your weight is over a size 16, for example, go find a challenge that will give you the tools, push you beyond your limits so that you do things you did not know were possible, and enable you to finally live the life you dream about. (FYI, I can help you with the last one, with a programme called The Weight is Over and if you want more information, visit my website: **www.chris-marcoflores.com.**)

Go back to the challenge task on page 189 and complete the task.

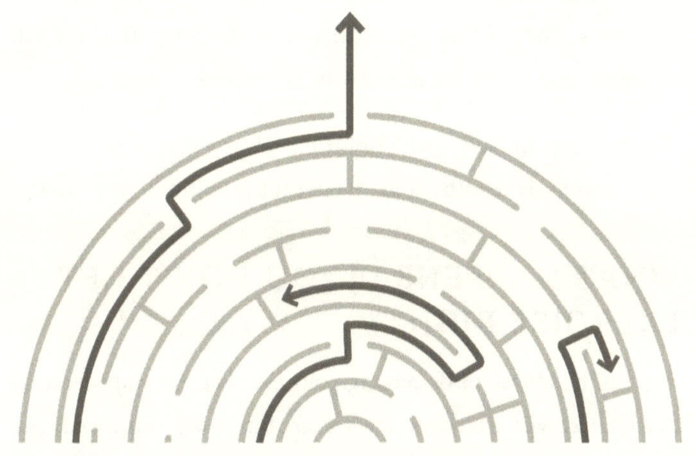

# VITAL ACTIVITY 3
## Exercise

## WHAT IS EXERCISE?

Exercise is an activity that requires physical effort to either sustain or improve your health and fitness. In this part, I am going to dive deep into exercise; however, I am going to explain how it needs to be combined with the correct nutrition.

# WHY IS EXERCISE A VITAL ACTIVITY?

Exercise is important because your body is built to move and it's a vital tool that enables you to look after your body. The more you look after your body, the better your life will be. It's like buying a car and never putting oil in it. If you never put oil in a car, sooner or later, your car will break down and you will never be able to use it because you never looked after it.

Exercising your body is like putting oil in a car, it keeps your mind and body healthy, and gives you the ability to stay agile.

# WHAT HAPPENS IF YOU DON'T GET EXERCISE RIGHT?

You can be at risk of damaging your body or not improving it, like Claire, who exercised for 4 years but never improved. She found it hard to escape an unhealthy, overweight body because she never included the right intensity exercise.

There are also a lot of people only doing the things they like to. For example, a normal exercise session should be broken down into sections, e.g. warm-up – main session – cool-down. Every single session should have a warm-up and cool-down. A lot of people skip warming their bodies up and jump straight into the main session instead. Because they are tired after their main session, they will skip the cool-down and just stop working out. If you do this you put your body at risk of long and short-term injury and put it under a lot of stress.

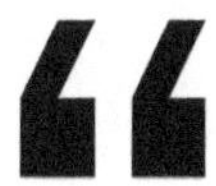

EXERCISING YOUR BODY IS LIKE
PUTTING OIL IN A CAR, IT KEEPS
YOUR MIND AND BODY HEALTHY,
GIVES YOU THE ABILITY TO STAY
AGILE AND MEANS YOU WILL NOT
BECOME FRAGILE.

# GETTING THE RIGHT ATTITUDE TO EXERCISE

If you are reading this and thinking, 'I do not enjoy exercise,' or 'I have no passion or desire to exercise,' then I'll guess the reason is either because:

1.  You have never been fit, so any time you do anything relating to fitness, you find it very hard and it's not enjoyable.

2.  You may be fit but still don't enjoy it. This is normally because you haven't found a type of exercise that you enjoy doing. For example, I know a lot of people who are fit go to the gym three times a week to lift weights, and yet hate it. The gym is not the only method to get fit. There are loads of options, like swimming, cycling, running, hiking, judo, boxing, rowing, climbing, roller skating, and dancing. You get the idea.

If you force yourself to do something you don't like, it will only be a matter of time before you give up.

However, in the very beginning you might have to force yourself to do something you don't enjoy until you reach a fitness level where other options are available (preferably, in the fit zone on my fitness level table). Then, once you are fit, spend the time exploring different fitness avenues; I promise you that you'll find something you love to do and exercising will become a part of your life.

You are built to move, walk, run, jump and climb, and if you can do so, you should take every advantage of doing so until that privilege gets taken away from you, as one day you may become too weak to enjoy doing it anymore! Some people are born without this privilege, so take advantage of it while you can.

## • EXERCISE CHALLENGE •

There are so many exercise challenges to do and it's hard to say which exercise is the best to start off with as every one of them is different. So I have created a challenge called the '30-Day Push-Up Challenge'. It doesn't matter if you cannot do 1 push up or can already do 50, I have created 7 different levels (1 being easy and 7 being very hard) and the aim of this challenge is to increase just 1 level in 30 days or increase the amount of reps you can achieve at your existing level.

### Step 1

Visit **www.chrismarcoflores.com**

### Step 2

Watch the video entitled '30-Day Push-Up Challenge'

### Step 3

Start and complete the challenge

# WHICH IS THE BEST EXERCISE TO ESCAPE AN UNHEALTHY, OVERWEIGHT BODY?

You literally have so many different ways you can do it. Each type of training is going to benefit you in different ways. A lot of people get confused when they try to work out which exercise is the best. You need to stop thinking like that because different exercise will give you different outcomes.

For example, people ask what is better, cardio or strength training? The answer is they will both benefit you. However, you will get different outcomes by only doing one or the other.

Cardio will help you to burn fat, but if you only do this, it will burn fat and muscle and that is why marathon runners look so skinny. So the outcome for most people is healthy but flat-looking muscles.

Strength training can be done in many different ways, with or without weights. It helps you to build muscle, and people who only endure strength training like lifting weights tend to have muscles that look full. For example, when you see men who have very big round biceps, it's probably because they spend a lot of time lifting weights. This normally scares a lot of women off, because they think they will have muscles like Arnold Schwarzenegger if they lift weights or do weight training and so they stay away from it. This is the wrong thing to do because the only way a woman can have muscle like male bodybuilders is if they enhance their bodies by using steroids or testosterone.

Remember the more muscle you have, the faster your body will burn fat. Any exercise, if performed correctly, will help you lose fat.

The way you want to lose fat is up to you. If you want to do it all from cardio you can, if you want to do it all from lifting weights in the gym you can do this also. What I highly recommend is to have a good balance of both and actively gain muscle whilst increasing your cardio fitness levels.

## EXERCISE IS A GREAT TOOL TO HELP YOU PUSH YOUR MIND

Use exercise as a way of learning to push your mind further than you can imagine! Learning to push yourself physically takes a lot of mental strength that helps build your mental strength, which is useful when you do things that are really mentally tough, like sticking to a nutritional meal plan.

Even pushing yourself to do very relaxed exercise sessions when you don't want to will help to increase your mental strength, and the bonus of doing a very relaxed and easy session is it's incredibly beneficial.

These could be sessions like walking for an hour or casually swimming for an hour or a nice gentle bike ride. These sessions will not only improve your mental strength but also your life because they help to release stress, aid recovery in your body, burn calories, release endorphins (one of the best forms of anti-depressant), just to name a few of the benefits.

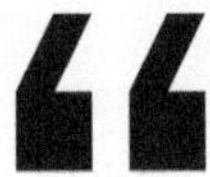

IF YOU ARE TRYING TO ESCAPE AN UNHEALTHY BODY, DON'T MAKE EXERCISING COMPLICATED OR TRY AND DO TOO MANY THINGS. IT IS IMPORTANT TO KEEP IT SIMPLE AND TO GET INTO A ROUTINE.

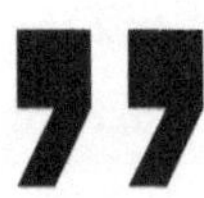

# WHEN DO YOU EXPECT TO SEE THE RESULTS OF EXERCISE?

If you train right with the right intensity, you will see results the same day! Yes, that's right, if you train right you will see results the very same day you train.

However, if you remain at the same intensity when you exercise, your body will start to become smart and adapt to what you are doing, and your progress will start to slow down or stop. That is why people see results very quickly when they first start working out, and it is easy for someone who is a size 22 to drop 3-4 dress sizes within the first three months.

If you want to continue to improve, you will need to increase the intensity. And from experience, it is quite good to change up the type of workouts that you do to shock the body.

Different exercises will use your muscle in different ways, and so when you change exercises you're changing the way you use your muscles.

As your body is not used to it, it will shock your body.

For example, if you spend six months trying to improve your running abilities and get to a level where you find it very easy to run and decide to change it up to a rowing session, I can guarantee that it will feel like your very first running session. After six months you may be at a good fitness level but you will be changing the way you use your muscles, so your body and mind will struggle throughout the session.

That's why military people are so fit, because they have such a dynamic training routine that ranges from gym sessions to outdoor running, obstacle courses, rack marches, mountain training, jungle training etc. The endless variety of training is the reason why they are in such incredible shape, both mentally and physically.

If you are trying to escape an unhealthy body, don't make exercising complicated or try and do too many things. It is important to keep it simple and to get into a routine, but it is always good to change your exercise routine regularly, so that you continue to improve.

√ Exercise TOP TIP

Never underestimate the importance of a warm-up and cool-down before and after exercise, it may add 10-15 minutes to your workout but it will give you 10 times the rewards when it comes to preventing injury and recovery. If you do not know how to do this, I have a warm-up and cool-down that you can do which is on my website: www. chrismarcoflores.com

## Progress in stages

You have to be very careful because if you are new to exercising, or have not exercised for a long time and find a very intense fitness session/class or personal training session so hard it makes you sick, then there is a very big chance it could put you off exercising. Even if you leave the session with the intention to go back, you'll find a reason not to go to the next session, even if you are all ready to go, and so will end up skipping it. Only a small percentage of people can handle extremely tough training right from the beginning.

I have been very guilty of this in the past by pushing clients who have never exercised in their life harder than was needed and they have never returned as a result. This, unfortunately, put them off fitness. Luckily, I learnt very quickly about the importance of progressing through the different levels of fitness and to make sure that I started at the relevant level. I have broken these down into 4 fitness levels with Level 1 starting with walking. All my clients tell me how lovely I am in the first two weeks and then, after the initial stage, I turn into a mini Hitler!

## THE 4 LEVELS OF EXERCISE

**Level 1** – Ease yourself in

**Level 2** – Increase the intensity

**Level 3** – Fear the session

**Level 4** – Find something you love

## Exercise Level 1: Ease yourself in

**Easing yourself in** can take up to 3 weeks.

**The objective is** to get your body and mind used to training for 5 days a week (preferably an hour at a time). These exercises are relatively easy.

It doesn't matter what kind of exercise you do, keep the intensity low. It is as simple and easy as that. You don't have to sweat, you just need to learn to keep moving for an hour.

The idea is to let your body know that you are going to be moving for 1 hour a day 5 days a week. The more you do this, the more your body will be prepared to progress to the next level.

## *How do you do this?*

I recommend just picking one of the three following exercises:

1.  Walking

2.  Cycling

3.  Swimming

Pick which days you are going to do this on and what time. If you are very new to exercising and find 5 days too hard, start off by doing 3 days, and then 4 the following week, and 5 the third week. However, if you can do 5 from the first week, I would recommend that.

Remember, the aim is to keep moving for 1 consecutive hour. However, if you are new, it may look a little like this:

Monday – Walk 10 minutes, rest 3 minutes – walk another 10 minutes, rest another 3 minutes, and repeat this for an hour.

7 days later – Walk 20 minutes, rest 2 minutes (repeat for an hour).

7 days later – Walk 30 minutes, rest 1 minute (repeat for an hour).

It is the same concept if you cycle or swim.

Each week you increase the exercise and decrease the rest. Ease yourself in.

When you start out, this will count as your main session but as you become fitter you will use this kind of session as your rest session.

## Exercise Level 2: Increase the intensity

**Increasing the intensity** can take 4-6 weeks depending on your abilities. Level 2 exercise sessions are not easy.

**The objective is** to be able to keep your heart rate elevated or in a zone known as the fitness zone for up to an hour. Now that your body and mind are used to exercising, you want to focus on increasing your fitness levels with a combination of cardio and strength and conditioning. Again, you will still want to aim to exercise 5 days a week, but 3 of the days will be Level 2 exercise sessions and 2 days will be Level 1 exercise sessions. As Level 2 exercise sessions put a lot of stress on the body, the

Level 1 sessions will act as recovery sessions and help the body to heal. These 2 levels of fitness are a great way to start building your fitness foundations.

## How do you do this?

This is slightly more complex as there are more options to choose from than in Level 1. You'll need to pick a type of cardio and strength and conditioning session that will elevate your heart rate consistently throughout the whole session.

Take a look at the list below for some ideas:

- Running (Cardio)

- Spinning (Cardio)

- Most fitness classes offered at most health facilities:

  - Pump (Strength and conditioning)

  - Circuit classes (This can be a mix of cardio, strength and conditioning)

  - Kettlebells (Strength and conditioning)

  - Boxercise (Strength and conditioning)

- Rowing (mix of both)

IF YOU TRAIN RIGHT WITH THE RIGHT INTENSITY, YOU WILL SEE RESULTS THE SAME DAY!

When you first start you may only be able to do 5 minutes at a time and then need to rest for 20 minutes between each 5-minute burst, but as the days and weeks progress, you'll want to push yourself. Even if you only increase this by 2 minutes each session, you will be amazed how quickly your fitness levels increase.

Within the The Weight is Over programme, I've created workouts you can do at home or in a gym that will accommodate Level 2. For more information, go to my website: www.chrismarcoflores.com

## Exercise Level 3: Fear the session

**Fear the Session** can take a little while. It's hard to put a time frame on Level 3 because you must stay at this stage until you have hit the goal you are happy with. It took me 6 months at this stage before I fully changed. It can take people up to 12 months as Level 3 exercises are challenging.

**The objective is** to train at a level where you are consistently improving. You don't want to adapt and remain the same. It's a very good sign when you take on a session and it gives you a slight feeling of fear because you know it is going to be hard, as this shows you are training at a level where you will improve.

Once you can keep your heart rate at the fitness zone level for an hour you move on to Level 3, and your recovery sessions will become a mixture of Level 1 and 2. As you become fitter, things change. For example, when you first start, jogging could be a Level 3 activity, but after working out for a few months, you may be able to do a light jog at Level 1.

You will still aim to exercise for 5 days a week, and want to do between 3-5 days a week of Level 3 and make the rest up of recovery sessions with Level 1 and 2 sessions. For example, in one week, you might do:

- 3 x Level 3 on Monday, Wednesday and Friday.

- 1 x Level 2 on Tuesday.

- 1 x Level 1 on Thursday.

## *How do you do this?*

Okay, here's the best way to understand this. You should aim to achieve more than you did the previous session. For example, if you chose to do running for your cardio and weight training for your strength and conditioning, your aim is to do better than the last session.

For example, if you can only run 4 miles without stopping then run 4.5 miles without stopping in your next session or if you ran 4 miles in 30 minutes, then your aim should be to run 4 miles in 28 minutes, which means you have to push yourself in both cases.

If your strength and conditioning session includes squatting with a 20kg barbell for 10 repetitions and 3 sets, your next session would be squatting 22.5kg for 10 repetitions and 3 sets or squatting 20kg for 10 repetitions for 5 sets, instead of just 3. (This would also depend on your workout programme.)

As you can see, you are doing more than the last session and that is how every session should be. This applies to all methods of training.

If you train right with the right intensity, you will see results the same day!

You should be in a strong enough state of mind and your WILL-POWER should be strong enough to fear the session. What I mean is that you have a slightly scared feeling in your stomach before the session even starts because you know it is going to be a tough session. But once you have finished the session, you will be pleased that you have done it.

The good news is you get to a certain point where you actually enjoy this feeling and look forward to pushing your body's limits, because the feeling you get after the session is indescribable and very addictive.

## Exercise Level 4: Find something you love

**Find something you love** that is ongoing.

Once you have reached your goal and are happy to maintain it, **the objective is** to find some sort of exercise that you love and look forward to, so that exercise no longer feels like a chore! It turns into a passion instead.

When people think of exercise, they think very small and only about options they have in the gym or something like running. But the options are endless, like tennis, rugby, football, boxing, dancing, swimming, hockey, triathlon training, basketball, pole dancing, MMA, hiking, and fitness classes. The list goes on. There are hundreds of different ways to exercise. There is one for everyone, you just have to find it.

You may not enjoy the previous steps (Level 1-3) but you must stick at them until you have reached your goal. Although there are some types of exercise that you love from the beginning, some exercises should not be done to get fit because they require a high level of fitness to begin with.

For example, MMA is an incredibly tough sport and if you started it when you are at Level 1, there is a very big chance it might put you off exercising completely. Remember, I said only a small handful of people can hack and endure tough physical exercise from the beginning. Unless something like that offers beginners training, stick with the method I suggested.

## How do you do this?

First, look at the options available to you locally. What sounds like fun? When you are trying to find something you love, you must give it some time (roughly 2-3 months) before making a decision as to whether you should give it up or carry on. For example, if you went to your local rugby or netball club to try these sports out, you are unlikely to be the greatest player on day one and may initially find it hard to enjoy because you are no good at it.

After a while, you develop the skills and you will be able to catch the ball and score goals or tries and then realise that you really enjoy it. Or you will be in a position where you are fit enough to play rugby or netball and have developed enough skills to play it, but still not like it. That is when you search for another avenue.

This relates to all types of exercise, even things like squatting with a barbell on your back, which is pretty much like sitting down and standing up. This might sound boring to some people but there is a skill to something as simple as that and a lot of people who gain it start to enjoy the art of being able to squat with heavy things on their back.

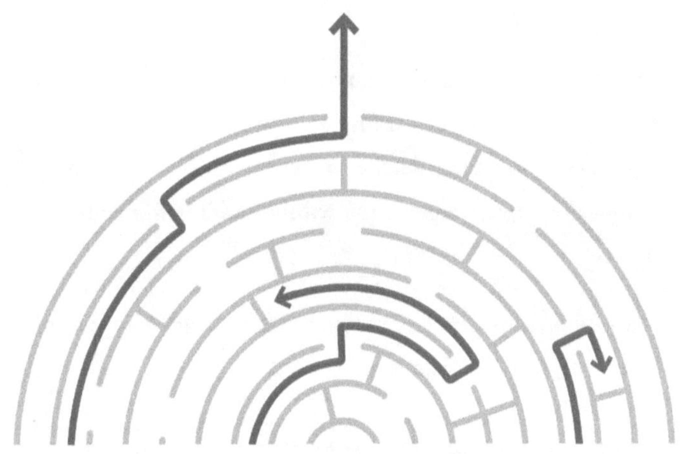

# VITAL ACTIVITY 4
## Nutrition

## WHAT IS NUTRITION?

Nutrition is fuel because what you put in your body will determine how you perform. It is kind of like a fire. If you put a sheet of A4 paper on an open fire it will go up in flames very quickly; however, the fire would die down very quickly. This is like putting poor quality nutrition in your body that only keeps you going for a short time. When you put a thick piece of wood on the fire, it takes time to burn and the fire remains alight for a lot longer. This is like putting high-quality nutrition into your body that keeps you going for a long time.

## WHY IS NUTRITION A VITAL ACTIVITY?

There is a great saying that you can't out-exercise bad nutrition, which means if you are trying to escape an unhealthy, over-weight body, no matter what exercise you do you will remain in an unhealthy, overweight body without addressing your nutrition.

Nutrition is a vital activity because you must get your nutrition right if you want to change.

## WHAT HAPPENS IF YOU DON'T GET NUTRITION RIGHT?

You may have heard this before, but nutrition contributes to the biggest percentage of the results you achieve. So if you get your nutrition wrong, you will only achieve a fraction of your desired result.

For example, if you are a size 22 and you want to become a size 10, nutrition can contribute 60% - 85% of your results. The rest will be made up of the type of exercise activity/programme that you combine with it.

# HOW CAN YOU FIND A SUSTAINABLE NUTRITION PLAN?

People are told they must do a nutrition diet they can sustain. This is true; however, trying to find a diet when you first start your fat-loss journey can be a slight problem. Let me give you an example.

This relates to both sexes but, let's say that Sarah, who has been a size 22 for the last 6 years, is sick of being in a body she is unhappy with and desperately wants to be a size 16.

Now for Sarah to change, things in her life must also change, which will disrupt her current lifestyle for a while, until she adapts to her new lifestyle.

As we are talking about nutrition, let's say that Sarah eats 4 large pizzas every single day. For her to lose fat, she will need to reduce the amount of calories she is currently eating. Now we know that Sarah likes to eat pizzas, so if we put pizza on her fat-loss diet, we can create a diet that Sarah can sustain, right? Well…

For Sarah to lose fat, she needs to reduce the amount of pizza she eats, and instead of having 4 large pizzas every day she can only eat 2. Great, but have we created a diet that Sarah will be able to easily sustain?

Well no, because she is now disrupting the lifestyle she is currently used to, and even though she is eating what she likes, she's not eating as many as she normally does. As a result, Sarah will find it hard to eat only 2 pizzas a day when she has been used to eating 4, and so now it becomes a diet that is hard to sustain. It will take some time before Sarah's body adapts and gets used to only eating 2 pizzas a day and not 4. Of course, that is just an example, I wouldn't advise eating pizza every day.

So, if you really want to change, you might need a diet which is hard to sustain (initially) even if it includes the foods that you enjoy. This is just until your body adapts to your new lifestyle.

## WHY IS IT SO HARD TO STOP EATING PROCESSED FOOD?

When you are hungry, your body craves nutrition, not food. When you eat processed food, your stomach will be full but your nutrition levels won't have increased. That is why you will want to snack very soon after eating something that is processed. When you eat food with good healthy nutritional value it raises your nutrition levels, which means you will be fuller for longer because your body has a good level of resources to use.

## WHY IS IT SO HARD TO CUT DOWN FOOD INTAKE?

Even if you eat only healthy foods, but eat more than necessary, your calorie intake may be too high. Your body will adapt to this high level of food and get used to it. When you try to cut down to a normal level, your body will tell you it's still hungry and needs more, until your body adapts.

# WHY DO I NEED TO COMBINE NUTRITION WITH EXERCISE?

People who only focus on one of the activities and not on the other lack balance. For example, it's very common to see a rugby player who is obese, yet they have very high fitness levels and no problem keeping up with the skinnier players on the pitch. This is because they will focus a lot of energy on increasing their fitness levels but completely disregard their nutrition.

These "fit and healthy" rugby players neglect their nutrition, and that is why they are obese. They also tend to have health problems that are related to being overweight, for example, heart problems, high blood pressure, high cholesterol, to name just a few.

My dad was this person. You couldn't have met a fitter rugby player. It somehow didn't look right to see my dad, an overweight man, running rings around the more athletic-looking players on the pitch. However, his downfall was that he neglected nutrition. He suffered from very bad heart problems and needed keyhole heart surgery, but couldn't have it because his blood pressure was so high. He had to lose a lot of fat before they could even consider operating on him.

Now you're probably thinking, I am a personal trainer and I specialise in helping people escape an unhealthy, overweight body they feel trapped in, why would my dad be overweight?

I always encouraged him to lose weight, but because he was so fit, he was blind to his health problems. He didn't listen and wanted to continue to enjoy his life by eating junk food regularly, until he was presented with the bad news about his heart. It was only then that he wanted my help.

We can flip this. It's also very common to see people who are very healthy with their nutrition but completely neglect exercise. These people are very healthy on the inside but can be very brittle and fragile because you build muscle that protects your body when you exercise. If there is no muscle to protect your body then it is at risk to any sudden impacts.

So those two little examples show you that it's important to combine both of them and not to do one without the other.

There are so-called health coaches out there who will tell you that all you need is nutrition, and encourage very little or even no exercise, which blows my mind.

Exercise and nutrition are two complementary parts of one whole! Like a knife and fork! Tea and biscuits! Pancakes and syrup! When one element is combined with another you have a far better outcome.

If you are trying to become a healthier person and your coach tells you to do one without the other, then find a different mentor/coach.

> **WHEN SOMEONE COMES TO ME TO ESCAPE AN UNHEALTHY BODY, IT IS MY MISSION TO TEACH THEM WHAT I AM DOING TO THEM SO THAT I CAN GET THEM TO A POSITION WHERE THEY WILL HAVE THE KNOWLEDGE TO DO IT WITHOUT ME.**

Anyone who has a good balance of both will back me up when I say that if you exercise right, you feel great after every session, and then if you replenish your body with good nutrition, it makes you feel on top of the world. Sometimes you feel like a mini superhero!

Just imagine what it would be like if this became your daily routine – having a great workout before your day even starts, and then spending the rest of the day filling your body up with nutrition that makes you feel amazing.

You don't need to be a genius to understand that is a recipe for a good life.

## GET IN THAT KITCHEN

In life, it's okay if you do not know how many stars there are in the sky or how deep the ocean is or how to fix an aeroplane, or who's number one in the singles charts. But some things in life are vital.

Like cooking. I meet so many people who say they can't cook and do not know how to. If this is you, think about it, you are going to be eating every day for the rest of your life! It might be a good idea to learn to cook. It's really not that hard.

Now, I am no Gordon Ramsey or Jamie Oliver, but I can make good, healthy, delicious food. Once you learn how to cook, it's easy to experiment with your own types of meals. It will give you the power to know how to exchange the bad food for the good. Meaning that instead of heading for McDonald's you can happily cook homemade healthy burgers, which can be much tastier than a McDonald's.

There are other essential things people dismiss in life that they should learn. As you are going to be eating every day, it is a good idea to learn what certain foods, drinks, spices and herbs do for your body. This is one of the best things you can learn, so that you don't just blindly buy into a diet plan without understanding what those foods (or the lack of those foods) will do to your body.

When most people pay for a personal trainer, they want to just turn up, do as they are told, eat what they are told to eat and turn into the person they desire. Then, as soon as they stop going to that trainer, they don't know why they've done it all and so end up going back to the person they don't like.

When someone comes to me to escape an unhealthy body, it is my mission to teach them what I am doing to them so that I can get them to a position where they will have the knowledge to do it without me.

## A WARNING ON UNDEREATING

It is not good to undereat. If your daily allowance of calories is 2,000 calories and you cut your allowance drastically to 600 calories a day, yes, 100%, you will lose weight but you are putting yourself in a dangerous position because you are having so few calories you are not giving yourself enough energy to survive. You will quickly become, grumpy, tired, unhappy and you will envy other people who are eating. And what happens when people undereat? As soon as they break their seal of 600 calories they end up binge eating and completely going off-track. The willpower it will take to get back on track to eat only 600 calories again is extremely hard and a lot of people never do.

There is no need to cut down to such a small number of calories. Most of my clients tell me I allow them to eat too much yet they get great results.

## NUTRITION PLANS, NOT PLAN

There is a reason as to why I encourage people to go through more than one nutrition plan. The majority of diets out there will work. As long as you have the formula right, it will work. I can't imagine how confusing it could be for people who don't know much about nutrition. I am a personal trainer with a lot of experience who is still forever researching new diets and their methods and I still get confused because of the amount of information that's available.

## NO ONE PLAN FITS ALL

I've mentioned this a lot, but I'll say it again: you cannot have one diet that is going to fit everyone in the world. Your friend might have done a diet, which did absolute wonders for them. It may do the same for you or it may not. All you know is that your friend's body responded very well to that particular diet.

A great saying that I always say to my clients is:

"You can give someone nuts and it's going to nourish them, or you can give someone else nuts and it will kill them as they are allergic to them."

Most diets out there will work and help you to escape an unhealthy, overweight body if they are done correctly. Each diet is built up of different methods, for example, some diets require that you only eat once or twice a day. If you are someone who enjoys eating lots of times throughout the day this is going to be a really hard one for you. Other diets will make you eat a high percentage of fats and a very low percentage of carbohydrates. If you are someone who enjoys eating carbs, this will also be a hard one for you.

I encourage my clients to try different diets and spend enough time with the diet so that their body adapts to it and, after a little while, my clients will find the diets they like and the methods they enjoy.

On my **The Weight is Over** programme, I take people through different diets. Most of them are 4 weeks long, some are 1 week long, others are 6 weeks. The allotted time for each diet is enough time for your body to feel the full benefits of that particular diet. Some are going to work extremely well for you and others not so much.

By doing this at the end of **The Weight is Over** you will not only know which diet works best for your body, but also your lifestyle (after your body has adapted, of course). This will be the diet that does not feel like a chore and you will be able to naturally maintain.

You should do the same. Figure out how well a diet responds to your body and, even when you do not like the diet, make sure that you ride it out until the end, because 6 weeks of your life will not kill you. It is the best way to understand a diet and you never know, you might surprise yourself and even love it by the end. This happens a lot. People think they don't like a diet and yet, by the end, it becomes their new diet for the rest of their life.

## ✓ Nutrition TOP TIP: food

The best way to stick to a nutrition method is to plan every single meal 4 weeks in advance, and then prepare your meals 7 days in advance. This means cooking all your meals on a Sunday ready for you to eat throughout the week. The clients who try to wing it and cook it along the way will fall off-track and break their nutrition plan 9 times out of 10. Stack the odds in your favour.

When it comes to nutrition, I highly encourage that you prep 7 days in advance. Learn to prep and create a habit of preparing. It will save you time and make it a lot easier to stay on track.

If you don't prep your food in advance, you risk eating the wrong things. From experience, if you've finished work and come home late and need to eat but you haven't prepared anything, the last thing you want to do is spend hours in a kitchen cooking food. A lot of people take the easy option and order ready-made food. However, if you've already had your healthy meals prepared in advance and all you have to do is take it out of the fridge and heat it up, it massively increases your chances of success.

Yes, I understand you need to enjoy your life, but if you are serious about losing fat, then you are going to have to stay mentally strong and stick to the healthy foods you have prepared for a period of time. Spending a year being careful about what you eat is much better than living a life of misery in a body you do not enjoy.

The clients I've trained who have not prepared their food, got either very small results or no results at all. Then they ended up blaming me, saying that the plan was just not working when really the issue was their lack of self-discipline about preparing food and sticking to a meal plan.

## PROGRESS IN STAGES

As with exercise, I have broken nutrition down into 4 levels. Why? Because if you have never lifted a weight in your life you wouldn't go into a gym and try to bench press 200kg. You would start at a weight you could do which might be as little

"

INCREASE THE NUTRITIONAL
VALUE. THIS CAN TAKE 4-6 WEEKS.
YOU WILL STILL BE BURNING FAT
AT THIS STAGE BUT IT'S A SLOW
PROCESS UNTIL YOU HAVE A
SUDDEN SPELL OF FAT LOSS.

"

as 10kg, then the following week this would increase to 20kg, and so on until you are strong enough.

Nutrition is the same. Going straight from a very bad processed diet to Strict Rick's diet is a recipe for disaster. Psychologically, you're going to find it very tough and it will only be a matter of time before you cave in. If it's very strict, it could put you off. Only a small percentage of people have the mindset to go from a poor diet to a strict diet.

Now, I completely agree that you can go from a poor diet to a good diet very quickly, but you must do it in the right way, and I believe that is one level at a time. Just like with exercise, you must ease yourself in and then progress through the levels if you want to be able to get through the journey.

## THE 4 LEVELS OF NUTRITION

**Level 1:** Get motivated

**Level 2:** Fill your levels up (increase the nutritional value)

**Level 3:** Manipulate your diet

**Level 4:** Turn it into a lifestyle

## Nutrition Level 1: Get motivated

**Get motivated.** This can take as little as a week. I believe the best way is to get quick results because it shows you that it is working and helps you start on a great path. Just remember though, this is only the beginning. What I do with all my clients is put them through a 7-day detox.

**The objective is** to give people quick results to motivate them to continue to do better. Even though they understand that this is a long-term thing and not a short fix.

## How to do it?

I put all my clients through a nutrition plan that I created called the 7-day detox. It is a tough plan to follow but it helps to decrease sugar and caffeine cravings and pushes a lot of toxins out of the body. It energises you, so not only will you see a visible difference in your body within just 7 days, but your body feels like it's been given an inside wash, which makes you feel amazing.

It also primes you for the next level, making it easier to stick to the regime.

## Nutrition Level 2: Fill your levels up (increase the nutritional value)

Increase the nutritional value. This can take 4-6 weeks. You will still be burning fat at this stage but it's a slow process until you have a sudden spell of fat loss. Then you will hit another slow stage and that is when you go to the next level.

**The objective is** to transition you from poor nutrition to good nutrition, so the nutritional value of what you fuel your body with increases. You will feed your body what it needs to work

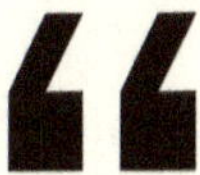

TURN IT INTO A LIFESTYLE,

THIS IS ONGOING.

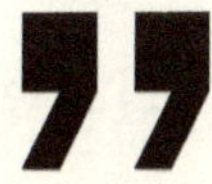

well and prime your body physically and mentally. Your body will be receiving all the nutrition it needs to function properly and, in return, it will provide you with enough energy to aid you through your exercise levels.

## How to do it?

I have created a nutrition plan called 'Keep It Simple', which does just that. I list all the ingredients that you can pick from and break them down into a list of fats, proteins, carbohydrates, and vegetables. It is a very simple method.

What you do is create three meals for the day by picking one or more ingredient from each list for each meal (in the plan, it explains how many you should pick off each list) and it is as simple as that.

You do this for six weeks, and after that, as long as you have been combining your nutrition with the relevant exercises, you will notice the difference and your mind and body will be ready to go to the next level of nutrition.

## Nutrition Level 3: Manipulate your diet

Manipulate your diet. It is a hard one to put a timeframe on because, for some people, the diet they pick will fit into their lifestyle perfectly and the only thing they will need to do is manipulate the amount they consume as they improve. Other people can try as many as 8 nutrition methods before finding one.

**The objective is** to not only escape an unhealthy, overweight body but also find which diet method works best for you and your lifestyle so that it provides long-lasting results. If you have a specific goal in mind, for example, going from a size 22 to a size 10 in 18 months, then it's important to manipulate your diet so that you can get predictable results. That way you will know exactly how much you have to lose each week and will actually do so.

## How to do it?

You can calculate every diet method to get the results you desire. This is the easy bit, finding one that your body works best with is the hard bit.

For example, 1lb of fat = 3,500 calories. If we reduce 3,500 calories from your weekly calorie allowance, you will lose 1lb of fat within that week.

However, your body will respond better and provide you with more energy if you consume wholefoods over-processed foods, but some foods will work better for you than others do.

It's just like the nut analogy. I can give one person nuts and it will nourish them and I can give someone else nuts and it will kill them. This is why we have to figure out which nutrition method and foods respond best with your body.

The best way to get to know this is to try and test different methods (don't let anyone tell you there is a one-size-fits-all diet). Experiment with some of the diets listed below, which are just some examples. Each one will aid different people. Some people like to eat 6 times a day, some only twice, some like to eat carbs, some don't. There is a method for literally anyone and everyone's lifestyle.

**The keto diet** is a high-fat low-carbohydrate method. Instead of burning carbohydrate for fuel in your body, it will burn fat.

**Carb cycling** is a diet in which you have a low amount of carbs for a certain amount of days and then replenish them with what some people call refeed/high carb days. There are lots of different ways you can do this. It could look like this: low carbs for three days and high carbs on the fourth, and then repeat this pattern. It's very well known that it will help your body to burn fat whilst not affecting your level of metabolism.

**Intermittent fasting** is a method where you will have a window with the number of hours you can eat in (this is normally an 8, 6 or 1-hour window) after which you must fast. If it is an 8-hour window you will have to eat all your food within these 8 hours and the same goes for 6 and 1 hours. (Again, there are a lot of different ways you can do this method.) When your body is not eating, your stomach is healing itself. So the longer you are not eating, the longer it is self-healing. Do not go and starve yourself. You must do this method tactically.

# Nutrition Level 4: Turn it into a lifestyle

**Turn it into a lifestyle, this is ongoing.**

**The objective is** to find the diet that does not feel like a diet (obviously after you have taken the time for your body to adapt) and something that you can naturally do without it feeling like a chore. This is your lifestyle diet. You need to keep this one going to help you improve in the long-term. When you get to this level, you will be able to get away with having a take-away every now and then, or consuming something unhealthy because most of your nutrition is healthy. One of the reasons why people find it so hard to escape an unhealthy body is because their life consists of so many bad habits, it's physically impossible to escape.

The aim is to change these bad habits to good habits to the point that it is impossible to be in an unhealthy body. That's right, it becomes impossible to be in an unhealthy body as you have turned it into a lifestyle.

I've created a video to help explain how you go from a lifestyle of bad habits to a lifestyle of good habits. It's called 'Change your lifestyle not just your diet' and is on my website: www.chrismarcoflores.com

## *How to do it?*

To do this you stick to a plan long enough for your body to adapt to this healthy lifestyle. It's a bit like the example I gave of Sarah, eating 4 pizzas a day.

Well, you want to adapt your body so it will crave more good nutrition than bad nutrition, so that 80% of your nutrition will be healthy.

## IT'S OKAY TO HAVE A CHEAT DAY, IT HELPS YOU STAY SANE

You will be able to incorporate a cheat day with every diet. You must make sure, however, that it doesn't conflict with the diet you are doing.

For example, if you are on a keto diet and the aim is to stay in ketosis, a cheat meal with lots of carbs would chuck you out of ketosis and jeopardise the whole diet. So make sure you understand what kind of cheat day you can have.

### Cheat day rule 1: mix it up

Just remember that having a cheat meal will become a habit, so you will need to be smart about it. Plan in advance when you are going to have your cheat day. If you have your cheat day on Saturday night, then your hormones will kick in every Saturday, ready for you to have your cheat day. And if you don't have your cheat meal you will get withdrawal symptoms. So, the way to do it is to make sure your cheat day is on a different day each week.

What happens when you mix it up? You'll disrupt your healthy eating and become so used to eating healthily that when it comes to the day that was supposed to be your cheat day, you'll start to lose interest because you would rather have the feeling of feeling good through eating good stuff.

## Cheat day rule 2: no alcohol, ever

Alcohol is the only thing that is not acceptable. I highly recommend cutting it out until you have hit your goal!

## Cheat day rule 3: plan it

Now notice how I have said cheat day! This doesn't mean you can sit down and have a conveyor belt of food going into your mouth all day! It doesn't quite work like that. You still will have to plan it.

I used to strategically plan one day a week. I would have a day where I would fill up on carbs, pizza, Chinese, burgers, you name it. Not all at once. I would pick one and strategically implement it into my diet each week. Amazingly, this method helped me to still enjoy what I liked once a week and get into the greatest shape of my life!

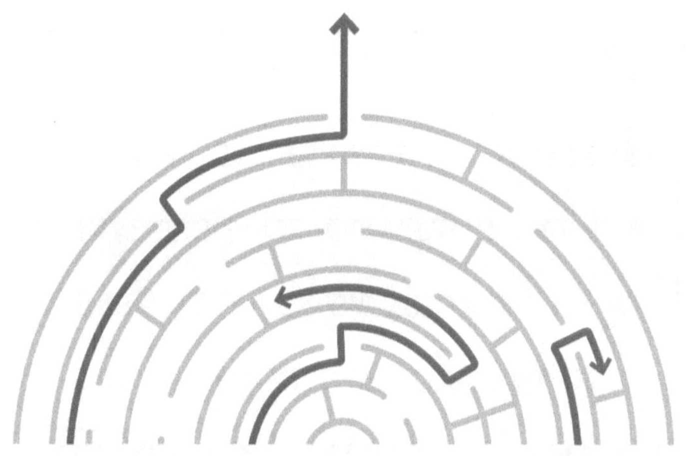

# VITAL ACTIVITY 5
## Planning and Preparation

### WHAT IS PLANNING AND PREPARATION?

Planning ahead will make you consciously aware of exactly what you are doing, and the more you plan the better your planning habits will be. At first, it may feel like a tiresome task. But it will turn into a habit.

There's one great saying that we were taught in the Army. It's called the 7 Ps – Proper Planning Preparation Prevents Piss Poor Performance. Anything in life that is planned works a lot

"MILLIONS OF PEOPLE THINK THAT ALL THEY NEED TO DO IS EAT WELL AND EXERCISE TO ESCAPE. WELL, THAT IS TRUE BUT IF YOU DON'T PLAN HOW YOU ARE GOING TO DO THIS, IT WEAKENS YOUR CHANCE OF ACHIEVING SUCCESS."

better than just trying to wing it. The longer you plan, the better the outcome. I have lived by this since my military days. Even when I was writing this book, I hired a coach to teach me what I needed to do and how to set it out. They spent a day with me to teach me what I should put into a book and why and how it should be laid out, by the end of the day I had a plan of what and how to write. I then used what they had taught me during that day and spent 2 weeks going through what we had planned to write in this book before I even put pen to paper, because, I wanted to be crystal clear about what I was doing and how I was going to do it. By doing this, writing the first draft of my book was simple. The only downfall was it was very time-consuming, tedious and mind-numbing because I am not a fan of writing in any shape or form. (That last paragraph was written during my first draft. I am currently on my third draft, and as I am re-reading this, I can relate my experience to people who do not enjoy exercising, and I often tell people the more they do it the more they will enjoy it. After I wrote the first draft the thought of going through it a second time killed me. However, I sent my first draft to a professional to check and they sent it back to me to correct. I took their feedback on board and now I really enjoy it and I am looking forward to going through the fourth and fifth draft).

Let me put that into perspective for you. I never finished school, so my writing ability is incredibly poor. However, I had the ambition to write a book and as you can see I have, with a lot of help.

Millions of people think that all they need to do is eat well and exercise to escape. Well, that is true but if you don't plan how you are going to do this, it weakens your chance of achieving success.

People who try and do this without any planning fail 9 times out of 10. They tell themselves they will start next Monday without any plan. Monday comes along and they wake up, have a healthy breakfast, or think they are having a healthy breakfast, go to work and have a healthy lunch, go to the gym and chuck some weights around until they are tired and leave.

If they haven't planned anything, they will either eat nothing when they get home, because they think that it is better than eating badly, or convince themselves that they have done so well that they deserve a glass of wine and then maybe a pizza. You may be able to relate to this.

Some people might do really well for a couple of weeks, and lose a bit of weight and feel good. Then, all of a sudden, they start adding in little treats here and there, and head back to their old lifestyle with its bad habits and end up putting all the weight back on again.

If you plan in advance, you will be setting yourself up to win because you will understand:

1.  What you are doing

2.  Why you are doing it

3.  How long it is going to take to achieve

4.  What you will need

To succeed, you need to carefully plan:

1.  What and when you are going to eat

2.  Where, when and how you are going to exercise

3.  What goal/challenges you are working towards and how you are going to achieve them

4.  How you will deal with temptation/obstacles

If you don't do each one of these, you will risk getting lost on your journey. For example, you decide to eat healthily, but you don't plan your meals, so you don't know what to buy when you go to the shops, or you plan to exercise during the week ahead, but don't plan when or what you are going to do. Therefore, come the end of the week, you may have not exercised once because you've had nothing set in stone as to what you were going to do. Each element is very important even if it does seem tedious.

## WHY IS PLANNING AND PREPARATION A VITAL ACTIVITY?

Anything you do without a plan is a risk. Imagine that you and your friends have jumped on a boat in New York and want to sail to Africa. You ask the captain if he knows where he's going, and he replies, 'Yeah, it's in that direction,' pointing out towards the ocean. All you can see as you look past his pointing finger is nothing but water and clouds. He has no map or compass. All he knows is the general direction.

Would you let him take you to Africa? Unless you're slightly crazy, not a chance in hell!

You would want to know:

- What boat he's using, and if that boat is capable of crossing the ocean.

- How long it will take, whether or not you need to bring food and water.

- Whether it has a built-in map and a radio that's connected to a control centre.

- If anyone on board has done this trip before.

That's a little extreme, so let's go for a lighter example, such as climbing a mountain.

You think it would be easy, right! Head upwards and you will reach the top! If you have never climbed a mountain, it is not that easy. You don't know whether you are going up or down on a lot of mountain paths (as mountains are not perfectly straight triangles, sometimes the land in a section of the ascent will gently decline before you reach your next climb). You can get lost very quickly. It is very dangerous.

You would want to have:

- The right equipment

- Emergency phones that will be able to reach you anywhere on the mountain

- Enough rations to last you the time of your duration

- A map and compass

Now for an even lighter example: a road trip across the desert.

But your car's fuel gauge is broken. Would you just jump in and hope for the best or would you want to make sure that you had enough fuel to get you to the next fuel station?

I'm pretty sure you wouldn't want to be lost in a desert.

All of these examples have one thing in common: if you don't plan properly, there is a very big chance of you getting yourself in a life-threatening condition. Being in an unhealthy, over-weight body increases your risk of potentially deadly health conditions, including:

- High blood pressure

- Type 2 diabetes

- Heart disease

- Stroke

- Certain types of cancer

- Osteoarthritis

- Fatty liver disease

- Kidney disease

That's only mentioning a few of the conditions that could hit you. The difference is that getting lost at sea, up a mountain or in the middle of the desert, and putting your life at risk, happens pretty quickly. Whereas putting your life at risk due to being overweight, creeps up on you over years of neglect and bad habits. But a lot of people only really take control when their condition becomes life-threatening.

## WHAT HAPPENS IF YOU DON'T PLAN OR PREPARE PROPERLY?

Without planning you will make bad choices. Let's say you are trying to tackle the nutrition side and you decide to go on a diet of healthy eating, but you are going to make it up as you go along. That is just a recipe for disaster. If you come home late from work and you have to be up early in the morning, and you are tired, stressed and you do not know what you are going to eat that night, the last thing you will want to do is cook. A lot of people end up going for the easy option and get a takeaway, I have even done this myself.

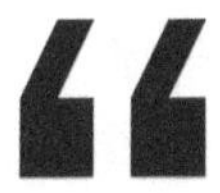

THERE WILL BE BOTH MENTAL AND PHYSICAL CHALLENGES INVOLVED IN LOSING FAT, SO IT IS BEST TO HAVE A STRATEGY FOR ALL THE POTENTIAL OBSTACLES THAT MAY CROP UP.

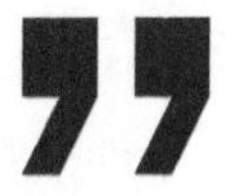

# PLAN FOR MENTAL OBSTACLES

If you don't know where you're going, you won't know what obstacles you are likely to encounter or have a plan that will help you deal with them.

There will be both mental and physical challenges involved in losing fat, so it is best to have a strategy for all the potential obstacles that may crop up.

For example, say you have been given a nutrition plan, so you know what you are eating but you do not know why you are doing it or what reaction you can expect from your body. When you start changing your body – losing fat – it will do everything it can to try and get back to where it feels most comfortable. Your mind will even try and tell you to stop doing what you are doing. You need to be prepared for this.

For example, if you are 280lb (126kg) and you lose 28lbs (12.6kg) through a diet, your mind will tell your body that it isn't normal to be at this weight. Your mind will start playing tricks on you. Have you ever been in a position where you can just eat and eat and eat, but never seem to be full? What happens is your mind flicks a switch in your head to tell you to keep eating because it wants you to get back to your normal level. It's not your body telling you it needs more fuel. Your mind can create all sorts of excuses when you start to change your body. Anything that you have stopped eating will look 1000x more delicious and tempting.

This is why knowledge plays an important part. If you plan in advance, you will understand why you are feeling the way you do when you hit certain hurdles and understand how to overcome them.

This is just the nutrition side, then you have exercise, barriers and challenges.

And if you are trying to escape an unhealthy, overweight body, you don't just plan once. You repeat the process every time you start a new diet or new exercise, and also when a new challenge or barrier comes into your life (which is roughly every 6 weeks).

## PLAN FOR TEMPTATIONS

Plan in advance how to handle your temptations, so you are prepared to fight them. You will come across temptations every day! Trying to consistently avoid them will be near on impossible, unless you send yourself to a camp where there are no McDonald's, Starbucks, all-you-can-eat Chinese, Thirsty Thursday night clubs, 2 for 1 pizza, cans of Coca Cola, the list goes on.

You are never going to be able to escape all the temptations, but the saying "out of sight, out of mind" will work to some extent. If you have a weakness for chocolate, removing all the chocolate from the house will make it physically impossible to eat chocolate at home. Unless you go out of your way to get chocolate.

# • PLAN TASK 1 •

## Step 1

Remove the temptations from your home. Go through your cupboards and donate whatever you shouldn't be eating to your local food bank (most supermarkets have a box you can add your donations to). You will be amazed how big your craving will be for something if you know it's sitting there waiting for you in the kitchen.

## Step 2

Go shopping and buy healthy snacks to replace the junk you will no longer be having. By planning in advance, you will have good healthy options available to you when you need them.

| Bad | Good |
| --- | --- |
| Chocolate | Nuts/Fruits |
| Coffee | Green, herbal, ginger tea |
| Crisps | Roast kale covered in olive oil (you can add seasoning to it, like pepper, ginger, and all sorts of spices and herbs). |
| Wine | A refreshing cold infused home-made flavoured water |
| Chinese | Homemade stir-fry |

| Bad | Good |
|---|---|
| McDonald's | Homemade beef burgers topped with cheese etc. |
| Brownies | Healthy homemade brownies |

The more you do this, the easier you will find it to say no when the temptation comes from an external source, e.g. a colleague who has brought in a tray of doughnuts to share.

## HOW TO PLAN

As the saying goes, there is more than one way to skin a cat! But you only need to learn and master one! (OH, that sounded good. I might have to patent that saying!)

It's so true though. Find a method and repeat it until it is engrained into your system to the point that it becomes second nature. My method has worked for me personally for over 10 years and unless someone comes up with something magical, I will be using it for many years to come.

When it comes to any health-related goals, such as losing fat, getting into shape or preparing for an event, you want to use this method. It keeps things simple and makes life easier for you as all you need to do is ask yourself these questions for each vital activity:

- What?

- Why?

- When?

- Where?

- How?

- How long?

## ✓ TOP TIP

You might think that planning and preparing will draw energy from you. Actually, planning and preparing will give you energy.

It's the same if you think about doing something; for instance, if someone thinks about doing something that will change their unhealthy lifestyle and lose weight but does not actually do it. This draws energy out of them, but if you are in an unhealthy, overweight body and you take steps to change your life, it will give you energy. A first step could be to talk to someone who can put a start date and a plan in place that is going to change your life and help you achieve the impossible.

It is as simple as that. When you know what exercise, nutrition and challenge you are doing, you can go into a lot more detail.

As soon as you veer off the plan and eat something bad instead of what you had planned, you will instantly feel guilty and it will make you want to get back on track.

It is the same with exercise. If you skip your planned workout, your body will be itching to get a workout fix in the day and you will find a way to make it work or make up for it another day.

## • PLAN TASK 2 •

## Plan your proven route to escape

*What*

| | |
|---|---|
| Mindset? | |
| Challenge? | |
| Exercise? | |
| Nutrition? | |

*Why*

| | |
|---|---|
| Mindset? | |
| Challenge? | |

| Exercise? | |
|---|---|
| Nutrition? | |

## When

| Mindset? | |
|---|---|
| Challenge? | |
| Exercise? | |
| Nutrition? | |

## Where

| Mindset? | |
|---|---|
| Challenge? | |
| Exercise? | |
| Nutrition? | |

## How

| Mindset? | |
|---|---|
| Challenge? | |

| Exercise? | |
| --- | --- |
| Nutrition? | |

## How long

| Mindset? | |
| --- | --- |
| Challenge? | |
| Exercise? | |
| Nutrition? | |

## TO FINISH OFF

Every great thing in life takes time; sometimes, it takes longer than expected to achieve these great accomplishments. As the saying goes, 'Rome wasn't built in a day.'

For example, when I decided I wanted to write this book, I expected to have it completed and published within 5 months. Yet, because writing does not come easily to me, and because I've had to spend time working with professional editors, it has taken me over 18 months to write and complete. But I got the help I needed and persisted until it was completed, even if it did take me twice as long as expected.

My point is, if you are in an unhealthy, overweight body and you want to escape, understand that it is unlikely to happen in just 6 weeks, or 12 weeks, or 6 months. It might even take 12 months or longer for you to fully escape, but it is not **Impossible.**

Another great saying that I love is:

*"Persistence beats resistance."*

Start your journey today and persist until you are in the position that you desire and turn your **The Weight is Over.**

# THE WEIGHT IS OVER: MAKING THE IMPOSSIBLE; POSSIBLE

**I** **have created** a programme that puts people through a fat-loss transformation to escape an unhealthy, overweight body that they feel trapped within. This is for people who have an unhealthy amount of body fat and would like to get into the healthy range.

What I do not do, is six packs, size zero or people who are looking to become Instagram models. I focus on helping people to feel comfortable in their clothes, to feel and look great every day and be confident to be able to take on any physical and mental challenge.

**My background** is in the British and American Army, where I completed extreme physical and mental challenges, and had the opportunity to learn how to master my mind and body at an elite level.

The military spends billions researching and understanding peak physical and health performance and all that research ends up in the hands of those in charge of getting soldiers into peak fitness, and of course the soldiers themselves. This was where I underwent my own personal transformation. This is where my passion to help others transform their lives was ignited.

I then become a personal trainer to further my learning and to create, test and develop my own methods that do not involve the screaming and the shouting but do get the same results..

My methods have allowed me to help 100s of people over the last 10 years to rapidly change their lives and the results speak for themselves.

- The last programme that I ran helped 41 people collectively lose over 1,400lbs (635kg) within 6 months.

- I have helped people who couldn't even think about jogging to the end of the road to complete a 10k mud run (within 6 weeks).

- I have transformed clients to the point they have been able to cancel gastric bands.

Just as important as the physical transformation is the confidence and energy I have helped my clients to regain.

64% of people are overweight or obese in the UK alone.[1] That's 3 out of 5 people who are suffering. This is very scary. What is worse, is this statistic is uncontrollably increasing in most western countries every single year. Are you a part of that percentage?

---

1 http://healthsurvey.hscic.gov.uk/data-visualisation/data-visualisation/explore-the-trends/weight.aspx

Most people understand what they need to do to lose weight. The problem is most people are now living lifestyles in which it is impossible to escape an unhealthy, overweight body. No matter what they do.

**In order to change,** and ensure you have long-lasting results, you need much more than just a diet plan. You need to understand what it takes to change your lifestyle, forever! And to be able to achieve this, there are some vital things that must happen.

My life experiences have helped me achieve a health and fitness level I didn't even know was possible. I now feel invincible to any physical and mental challenges.

When I see people who are at a poor level of health and fitness and do not believe it is possible to get themselves into the healthy zone it saddens me. I know if they were in my hands, I would change their life, forever. I get no greater joy than being the person who opens up someone's eyes and shows them what they do not think is possible, and ultimately **Making The Impossible; Possible.**

What I have created is not a quick-win plan. The results I get do not happen overnight. If you understand that it could take up to 12 months for you to lose weight and escape an unhealthy, overweight body that you feel trapped in, and you are happy to take on what will most likely be the toughest journey of your life, but one of the most rewarding, then see if you qualify to be one of the very few people I take on each year to go through my programme, **The Weight Is Over: Making the Impossible;**

**Possible.** If you would like more information and to apply then visit **www.chrismarcoflores.com.**

For some reason, people always ask if they could shrink me and keep me in their pocket and why haven't they found me sooner.

By the end, their lives are completely changed and they are able to do things they didn't think possible.

I hope you have enjoyed this book and if you are someone who wants to escape, hopefully we get to work together soon.

| Page number | Notes |
| --- | --- |
|  |  |
|  |  |
|  |  |
|  |  |
|  |  |
|  |  |
|  |  |
|  |  |
|  |  |
|  |  |
| Page number | Notes |
|  |  |

| Page number | Notes |
| --- | --- |
| | |
| | |
| | |
| | |
| | |
| | |
| | |
| | |
| | |
| | |
| Page number | Notes |
| | |